DATE DUE

OCT - 5 1993	NOV 1 8 1998
	OCT 1 7 2001
OCT 1 9 1993	NOV 3 0 2001
NOV - 1 1993	OCT 1 7 2004
NOV 1 5 1993	
NOV 2 9 1993	
APR 8 1994	
APR 2 0 1994	
APR 2 2 1994	
OCT - 6 1994	
NOV - 2 1994	
NOV 1 6 1994	
NOV 2 8 1994	
FEB - 6 1995	
MAR - 1 1995	
MAR 2 4 1995	
MAY - 1 1995	
AUG 1 5 1995	

Inside Nursing

SUNY Series, Teacher Empowerment and School Reform

Henry A. Giroux and Peter L. McLaren, Editors

Inside Nursing

A Critical Ethnography of Clinical Nursing Practice

Annette Fay Street

State University of New York Press

Published by
State University of New York Press, Albany

© 1992   State University of New York

For information, address State University of New York
Press, State University Plaza, Albany, N.Y. 12246

Production by M. R. Mulholland
Marketing by Bernadette LaManna

Library of Congress Cataloging-in-Publication Data

Street, Annette Fay, 1948–
       Inside nursing : a critical ethnography of clinical nursing
practice / Annette Fay Street.
             p.   cm. — (SUNY series, teacher empowerment and school
reform)
       Includes bibliographical references and index.
       ISBN 0–7914–0804–3 (pb : alk. paper) . — ISBN 0–7914–0803–5 (ch :
alk. paper)
       1. Nursing—Australia—case studies.   I. Title.   II. Series:
Teacher empowerment and school reform.
       [DNLM: 1. Nursing—Australia—case studies. 2. Nursing Staff,
Hospital. WY 125 S91451]
       RT15.S74   1992
       610.73'06'9—dc20
       DNLM/DLC
       for Library of Congress   90–10420
                                                                                    CIP

10 9 8 7 6 5 4 3 2 1

For Robert,
Benjamin, and Joel

Contents

❧

Foreword

Nursing is a strange occupation. It has many strengths and in general is practiced by a body of people who enjoy their work and who believe the work they do has an intrinsic value to society. If you ask all these very same people to explain their work, to explain what is "good nursing," to explain how they make judgements and decisions in their day to day work, most of them flounder. In recent years a great deal of time and effort has gone into encouraging nurses to think about theories of nursing, models of nursing that purport to describe nursing practice. Many registered nurses who care for people in hospital wards and departments have viewed nursing theories at best as being distant from their work and at worst as irrelevant. The use of the requirement for more systematic documentation has been viewed as a requirement of administration and not particularly relevant to what they, the nurses are actually doing. There has been, and still is, a gap between what we as administrators and teachers believe is needed to maintain and improve nursing care and how the practitioners view their work, their world of nursing practice. This is but one manifestation of the theory/practice gap.

Inside Nursing offers a very different way of viewing the theory/practice gap and a methodology that has potential to eliminate that gap. It is a seminal publication, which offers an exciting glimpse of what the future could be for nursing, for nurses, and for the community for whom nurses care.

Mary Patten
Deputy Executive Director
Royal Children's Hospital
Parkville, Victoria
Australia

Acknowledgments

This book represents a process of exploring clinical nursing practice. I did not walk the path alone, and so I would like to thank many others who have entered into the process with me or supported me through it.

Although unable to name all who have participated in this process with me, I would like to offer my special thanks to the following people who helped me and believed both in the project and in my capacity to complete it.

I begin by paying a special tribute to the constant love, inspiration, and care given to me throughout this project by my husband Robert and our sons Benjamin and Joel.

Thanks to John Smyth, who has challenged my capacities to think critically and rigorously, and who has patiently mentored me through the process of researching, writing, and reflecting, with encouragement and humor. Thanks to other staff at Deakin University who have listened and encouraged, particularly to Stephen Kemmis, a valuable friend. A special thanks to Cheryle Moss who gave generously of her time, knowledge, expertise, and hospitality.

Sincere thanks is due to the anonymous nurses who taught me about their clinical nursing practices and who shared themselves, their histories, their actions, their thoughts, and their values within the reflective process. I am also indebted to all those other nurses who talked with me, to the hospital researcher who acted as my sponsor, and to the administration of the hospital for the opportunity to conduct the research in the hospital.

Thanks also to Mary Patten, Andrew Robinson, and Kim Walker, my colleagues at the Royal Children's Hospital in Melbourne, who have the courage to share my vision and have demonstrated their faith in this book. Tony Stratford has provided excellent technical support while Judy Waters has shared of her publishing expertise.

This book would not have happened if it hadn't been for the persistent motivation and support provided by Peter McLaren, whose writing continues to be a source of delight and whose belief in my work amazes me.

Abbreviations

    As this document deals with nurses, and with their actions, excerpts from the data contain some of the more common abbreviations, which they use in their speech about, and reports of, their practices. However, throughout the research an attempt has been made to use nontechnical language when describing practices.

RANF:	Royal Australian Nursing Federation (Victorian Branch)
RN:	registered nurse
SEN:	State Enrolled Nurse
CN:	charge nurse .
ICU:	Intensive Care Unit
physio:	physiotherapist
blood gas:	the amount of oxygen and other gases in blood
RIB:	Rest in bed
Admin:	Nursing Administration (unless specifically identified as the hospital administration)
CCU:	Coronary Care Unit
CAG:	coronary artery graft
IV:	intravenous
O.T.:	occupational therapist

Introduction

In their propensity to acknowledge schools as the primary site of social and cultural reproduction, critical educational researchers have generally overlooked two important considerations. First, they have operated out of binary oppositions such as reproduction versus resistance which underplay the complex and contradictory play of power and practices at work in schools. Second, they have largely overlooked other important public spheres where pedagogy and power play mutually constitutive roles in the production of complex practices. In this important new work, *Inside Nursing: A Critical Ethnography of Clinical Nursing Practice,* Annette Fay Street not only provides a theory of cultural production that refuses to locate itself in the facile language of binary oppositions, but she also chooses as the setting of her study the neglected site of the metropolitan hospital. In this respect, *Inside Nursing: A Critical Ethnography of Clinical Nursing Practice* is a book that is long overdue.

Conducting her research in a large general hospital in Melbourne, Australia, Street's ethnographic work is one of the first large-scale studies of medical knowledge and nursing culture undertaken by a critical social theorist working within the tradition of critical and feminist pedagogy. It is a work that distinguishes itself in a number of important ways from previous research into nursing procedures and practices. First, in exploring the relationship between nursing knowledge and practice, it treats the production of meaning in its temporal, spatial, cultural, and historical situatedness. Secondly, as a study largely informed by feminist theory, it is critically attentive to the oral culture of nursing and the practical knowledge nurses utilize in their work. Street's analysis is primarily structured around how nurses themselves critique and contest medical domination, administrative structures, gender politics, and the hierarchies of power and privilege that devalue their clinical knowledge and practice. Within such a context, she is able to posit a type of knowledge which she calls "nurturance/knowledge" as both a critique and extension of Foucault's concept of "power/knowledge." This further enables her to challenge in a dialectical fashion the "power/knowledge" relationships at work in clinical medical settings. Thirdly, Street directly confronts the traditional view of nursing practices as an unproblematic site of harmony, consensus, and progress. Instead, she situates such practices within a culture of disjuncture, rupture, and contestation. In Street's analysis, the ideological dimension of medical transactions is not erased against the prevailing image of medical culture as a site of harmonious relations among doctors, nurses, and patients, on the one hand, and a caring an efficient pathway to health on the other. The culture of nursing is reclaimed in Street's perspective as a site in which the intersection of power, politics, knowledge, and practice give rise to a contested terrain of conflict and struggle.

Street is particularly adept as a researcher in her ability to bring to the reader insights which are couched in a profound respect for her research participants yet which challenge the very presuppositions which inform their daily pracitces. At the same time, she is prepared to locate her own practice as a collaborative researcher and medical worker, within structures of power and privilege that extend beyond the immediate social and institutional arrangements of the hospital setting. Furthermore, as a collaborative researcher and critical ethnographer, she acknowledges the interests served by her own ideological predilictions and in doing so disavows any claims to a master narrative or a privileged political discourse parading under the mantle of a universalizing truth. But unlike some feminist theorists, when Street disavows universalizing claims and affirms the epistemological virtue of partiality, she does not do so by refusing to locate herself within a political project in which she addresses concrete forms of domination and oppression. In this case, rather than disavowing the political, Street extends its implications by applying the notion of ideology critique to her own location as a historically and socially constructed cultural worker. In this instance, she does not succumb to a form of "white guilt" characterized by the newly fashionable assumption that no one but the most visibly oppressed have the right to speak. Instead, she "rages" against a history that both silences political agency and ignores the specificity of concrete struggles and the interplay of diverse social movements. For Street, the primacy of the political asserts itself not in speaking for others, but *with* others in relation to important social, political, and economic issues. One outcome of this approach is that Street is able to dismantle from the ground up, so-to-speak, the logic of positivism that informs the normative medical paradigm—a paradigm that is based on the male-dominated natural and physical sciences—and to provide directions for alternative practices that contest phallocentric power and standards of medical authority and a search for forms of nursing automony that refuse to emulate the logic of patriarchal domination.

Street's book challenges and unsettles the hierarchy of medical knowledge that reproduces its own privileged status by virtue of its ability to evoke a sanctifying presence, an aura of unproblematic authority that remains as unchallenged as the social conditions which it both mediates and produces. She is able to reveal the daily structuring of relationships of power and dominance between doctors and nurses in health care settings and explain how and why these both reflect and support relations of legalized medical dominance in the larger society. Her book asks the questions: What are the social consequences of the current gendered and technical division of labor within the medical profession in which doctors have privileged access to particular forms of medical knowledge and practices? Specifically, what does this mean for the deskilling and proletarianization of nurses in a medical culture that produces institutionalized forms of domination based on race, class, gender, and age?

Street makes it clear that to a large extent, the discourses of the medical establishment reproduce their hegemonic status by socially disguising their reproductive role in maintaining existing class, race, and gender relations that exist outside the various cultures of medicine. In part, she undertakes her analysis of the reproductive nature of the medical profession by demystifying and challenging the economies of power and privilege present in the structures and practices of clinical nursing which too often serve to produce what paulo Freire calls "horizontal violence" and "cultures of silence."

    Street's book is unique and pioneering in her treatment of clinical nursing as discourse-sensitive practices which possess both constraining and enabling possibilities for the historical agent. She is able to do this without privileging what Anthony Giddens calls the "imperialism of the subject" that he attributes to interpretive theory, and also the "imperialism of the object" which informs more totalizing theories such as structuralism and functionalism. In particular, Street takes up the challenge of how nurses are unwittingly complicitous in maintaining premataure closure on the discourses and practices open to them in their daily clinical practices that would enable them to escape the debilitating prejudgements of their inherited tradition and ultimately challenge and transform their professional roles as care givers.

    Street is acutely sensitive to the means by which nursing practices are devalued by forms of legislated medical dominance which serve as both social and scientific regimes of truth that authorize, naturalize, and legitimize nursing practices, providing an aura of clinical sanctity while at the same time camouflaging the relations of power that they support. She is able to reveal how the medical profession has colonized the definition of what constitutes legitimate clinical medical practice for nurses, and what knowledge should be of most worth, and sets forth cogent arguments with respect to why nurses should challenge the structured subservience that has all too often been the fate bequeathed to them by a logocentric, Cartesian-based exercise of male power.

    But Street does not restrict her analysis to forms of ideology critique, she also analyzes how power works to inscribe and contain the materiality of the body within clinical nursing practice. Hence, Street argues that "nurses are embodied people whose habitual bodily patterns and routines cause them to act in particular ways." By stressing the process of embodiment, Street is able to further the theoretical discourse of critique and possibility as part of a critical practice of nursing culture. More specifically, in taking up the issue of how power inscribes, contains, and produces habitual practices through various technical discourses and prescriptions, Street expands the terrain of contestation by including but moving beyond textuality to the materiality of social practices and the terrain of bodily practices (Giroux and McLaren, 1991). In other words, the process of embodiment helps Street to explain how nurses are positioned within the hegemony of a prescriptive technical approach to patient care which not only alienates the patients but also subjugates the nurses. Street vividly conjures up examples of how such practices are expressed. For example, Street writes that, for the nurses she observed, "it was quicker and less stressful...to continue to allow their bodies to work in ritualized ways than to act independently on the basis of a conscious decision, even when those actions could be demonstrated to contribute to the maintenance of technologies of power which were oppressive."

Yet for Street, power through embodiment is not simply oppressive but works relationally and dialectically to enable nurses to engage in proactive practices of ideology-critique and transformative praxis. In this regard, Street's work itself embodies what Anzaldua (1990: xvi) refers to as the "interface"—"the place...between the masks that provides the space from which we can thrust out and crack the masks." It is from this space that nurses are able, in the words of bell hooks (1990: 340), to engage in "talking back." For hooks, "Moving from silence into speech is for the oppressed, the colonized, the exploited, and those who stand and struggle side by side, a gesture of defiance that heals, that makes new life and new growth possible."

Following from this perspective is Street's recognition that nursing is more than a reproductive site for the accomodation of asymmetrical relations of power, for the perpetuation of patriarchy and internalized self-hatred among women, for the institutional silencing of largely female voices, and for other instruments of structural oppression. As powerful as the relations of domination are within clinical nursing practices, nurses frequently engage in a conscious refusal to become simply professional dupes. Instead, they participate in acts of resistance and contestation—acts of "interfacing" and "talking back."

Inside Nursing explodes the repressive myths of the cultural sites in which health care is practiced and produced. In reading her volume, we are provided with a language of counter-discursive possibility and transformation. Annette Fay Street's volume on clinical nursing practices appropriates critical social theory, critical pedagogy, and feminist theory not only as a means of interrogating the expansive hegemony of nursing practices in metropolitan centers of medical power but also as an attempt to develop more enlightened and liberating

health care practices. Street's study advocates a non-prescrip-
tive, broad-based theory developed from nursing and patient
experiences and opposes the prescriptive, formulaic, and technical application of knowledge which currently reproduces the
cultural basis of health and illness in Western societies. It is a
work that helps to both facilitate transformations in clinical
nursing practice and provide a transformative and health
enhancing environment by enabling nurses to analyze and
resist the hierarchical power and the ethical and technical
basis of dominative medical decisions. It is a work that, in our
estimation, will play a key role in the struggle for greater
automony among nurses.

Inside Nursing constitutes a profound, if disturbing, challenge to the hegemony of the health care system and should be
widely read by cultural workers in hospitals and school settings and by all those interested in developing conditions within our health care and learning institutions that further the
goal of social justice, an ethics of care, and on-going struggle
for human dignity and freedom.

—Henry A. Giroux and Peter L. McLaren

1

❦

Reflections on a Journey of Exploration into the World of Clinical Nurses

We shall not cease from our exploration
And the end of all our exploring
Will be to arrive where we started
And know the place for the first time.

T. S. Eliot, *Little Gidding* V 1944

My excursion into the world of nursing practice was a journey of exploration, a journey located in a specific time and context but which functioned as a revealer of fresh insights for myself and my colleagues who are nurses. I began this journey by posing the question:

How Do Nurses Think, Act, and Reflect on Their Clinical Nursing Practices?

To undertake this journey of exploration required me to make decisions about a theoretical basis that would inform and challenge the emergent understandings and an appropriate methodology with which to attempt to answer this question. I decided to examine clinical nursing practices from the perspective of critical theory and feminist critiques. In order to do this I, as the principal researcher, collaborated with four nurses working in an acute-care public hospital to engage in a critical ethnography, a research process that is openly ideological in design and emancipatory in intent. Through this collaborative process of inquiry, we systematically collected descriptive accounts of nursing action as a basis for theorizing and critique.

Nursing is an occupation that is female-dominated in constitution but has traditionally been subordinated to the male-dominated medical profession; likewise, clinical nursing knowledge has traditionally been subordinated to medical knowledge. Medical knowledge is generally treated as objective, value-free scientific knowledge, a view that mystifies both medical knowledge and the work of the doctors who use it. This view of the value of medical knowledge has been legitimated by the state through legislation, which accords specific responsibilities and rewards to doctors while legally subordinating the roles and responsibilities of other health professionals to them. This view of the medical knowledge as objective scientific knowledge is an apolitical view that disregards the ideological component of medical knowledge and the way in which it is exercised as social control to reproduce and support the class and gender interests of doctors.

Nursing has supported this apolitical view by its oversubscription to externally derived understandings of nursing developed through obsequience to the dominance of medical knowledge and practices. Historically, nurse scholars and educators have accepted the superiority of the technical knowledge of doctors by appropriating both the forms of knowledge and the paradigm in which this knowledge is created. Thus, they have unwittingly perpetuated the oppression of nurses and of their clinical nursing knowledge. Technical knowledge with its capacity to explain and prescribe is used by doctors and nurses as the basis for instrumental action. However, both doctors and nurses generally ignore the fact that this action is ideologically embedded within the sociocultural world of healthcare practices, which is subject to values, ethics, traditions, and the subjective and intuitive understandings of the healthcare practitioner.

The changed understandings of the roles and capacities of women within the community have been mirrored within the development of nursing knowledge. Critiques of the handmaiden role of nurses and the explication of the doctor/nurse game has led to a desire to develop nursing knowledge that is distinctive to nursing. This emphasis on the need to understand

and to describe and explain nursing practice has predominantly been taken up by nurses who have worked to develop objective, value-free knowledge about nursing practice. However, a growing emphasis has been upon the need to develop knowledge about the practical knowledge that nurses have and use in clinical nursing practice. This knowledge is subjective, value-laden, traditionally formed, and contextually embedded in the practices of clinical nurses. Nurses interested in developing this knowledge have focused on the development of meaningful intersubjective relationships between the nurse and the patient, which disclose the traditions, rituals, and pre-judgements that each brings to the situation. This process develops practical knowledge enabling nurses to make deliberate choices between alternative courses of action by subjecting their values, purposes, and commitments to scrutiny in the light of the constraints and exigencies of the situation.

This approach has provided nurses with valuable practical knowledge of the intentions and meanings of their nursing actions. However, it neglects questions concerning the relationships between the nurse's interpretations and actions and the structural elements of the healthcare situation. It enables nurses to examine intersubjective meanings but not the socially constructed reality through which these meanings are created and maintained. The focus is on clarifying individualized interpretations thus ignoring the power relations at work, which shape and form the consciousness of the nurse and patient and which are open to contestation as a form of false consciousness.

Feminist critiques of male-created roles and structures have informed critiques of the male-dominated medical profession and the implications of this dominance for nursing. Neo-Marxist and radical feminist analyses have begun to challenge the power relations at work in nursing as a basis for the development of alternative perspectives, which value the knowledge and experiences of women. However, these perspectives have not been generally well received by nurses because the analyses lead to alternate views of women's health issues and health practices, which develop alternate structures that bypass the medical system.

Nurses are beginning to recognize the need to examine the relationship between the manner in which power is experienced and exercised within nursing practice and the kind of knowledge that evolves from and informs this kind of analysis.

According to Perry:

> Nurses must discover ways to effectively challenge the taken-for-granted explanation that the individual is "responsible" while the system merely exists; and to challenge the taken-for-granted dominance of one form of knowledge over another, and one set of values over another. (Perry, 1987:9)

Through a commitment to feminist perspectives and the insights of critical social science, this research was an attempt to meet this challenge. In order to do so it was necessary to develop collaborative critiques of the forms of knowledge that are used in nursing practice and of the ways in which these kinds of knowledge serve particular interests. An examination of these interests can serve to uncover the power relations at work and the manner in which knowledge is socially constructed and ideologically embedded. This kind of analysis would have a deliberate and articulated agenda to develop an empowering and educative process in which nurses would be actively encouraged to reflect on their nursing actions, the understandings that inform them, and the contextual situation within which they work as the basis for transformation.

This reflective process facilitated an inquiry into the historical, cultural, and taken-for-granted meanings that informed nursing actions in order to disclose the interests being served by their continuance. Through critique we examined the relationships between power and knowledge and focused on the hegemony by which oppressive practices were maintained, accommodated, or resisted. Feminist critiques helped us uncover instances of transformative actions, which could not be analyzed using power/knowledge. This led to a recognition of the unspoken values of nursing practices, which differed from the explicit values espoused by nursing scholars interested in analyzing power relationships in nursing. These unspoken values led to emancipatory knowledge through an engagement in nurturance activities and helped to uncover the strengths and limits of critical social science for knowledge in nursing. The research did, however, demonstrate the potential for enlightenment, empowerment, and emancipation of clinical nurses through the pursuit of the dialectical relationship between power/knowledge and nurturance/knowledge.

The Politics of the Research Method

In beginning this research I took the view that nurses are not "cultural dopes" who are unable to participate in and contribute to a collaborative understanding of clinical nursing practice. Rather the research design was based on the premise that nurses think and act in meaningful ways within the rich tapestry which constitutes clinical nursing practice. However it was posited that these ways of thinking and acting need to be the subject of scrutiny and contestation in order to uncover the taken-for-granted habitual actions and the contradictions between intent, meaning, and action. This kind of critique endeavors to disclose the power relations at work, which perpetuate oppressive and hierarchical structures in nursing practice, and seeks to uncover the ways in which these power relations affect the daily lives of clinical nurses, constituting the limits and development of their clinical knowledge.

The research act was regarded as a political act because it assumes that nurses are capable of reflecting upon the processes of their own nursing practice, in the light of the processes of power relations, to uncover the ways in which they have unwittingly collaborated in their own oppression. The research process intended to bring about a transformation of nurses' understandings of clinical nursing practice and of their clinical actions. This approach is premised on the understanding that nurses not only collude in their own oppression but also engage in intentional oppositional actions in which they resist oppression and challenge hierarchical structures. The research examined the dialectic nature of some of these oppositional moments in order to highlight their potential for enlightenment and empowerment.

Collaborative reflection upon nursing actions, nursing understandings, and the socially constructed culture of clinical nursing practice was regarded as a methodological tool by which the researcher and the nurse participants can critique clinical nursing practice with an openly espoused agenda to facilitate emancipatory change in knowledge and action.

The Method: Critical Ethnography—A Collaborative Case Study

This study was designed to describe and analyze clinical nursing practice through the process of an in-depth long-term engagement in case studies of the nursing practice of clinical nurses. This engagement was based on the premise that an examination of nursing practices that attempts to challenge the contradictions in knowledge and action, which have been systematically distorted by history and ideology, will need to begin with thick descriptions of nursing actions. The choice of methodology stemmed from a belief that self-reporting of nursing actions and their meanings, a fashionable methodology in nursing research, ignores the problems of self-monitoring within the reporting process and the problem of false consciousness. By ignoring these aspects the researcher becomes open to the charge of rampant subjectivity, and under the guise of disinterested interpreter of the data, the researcher may perpetuate and legitimate forms of cultural oppression.

In order to procure these thick descriptions of nursing practice as a basis for collaborative analysis, I chose to engage in an ethnography, a comprehensive case study. Ethnography, like many methodologies, can be formed within different understandings of research and knowledge development, and informed by different knowledge needs. The kind of question posed determines the types of appropriate methodologies for consideration. Critical social science, with its capacity for the identification and analysis of issues concerning power and knowledge relations in the social order, poses questions in order that the exploratory research process itself is predicated upon a transformative focus towards knowledge and action. An ethnography framed within this context of critical inquiry, predisposed to rationally analyze and change unjust and irrational social activity, was classed as a critical ethnography in order to distinguish it from ethnographies with no transformative agenda whose purpose is framed to describe and interpret cultural realities.

A key component in any critical inquiry is the capacity for self-reflection and collaborative analysis to effect rational change. This process necessitates not only a reflexive relationship between the data and the researcher as advocated by Hammersley and Atkinson (1983) but also requires reflexivity with the research participants. This means that research participants have access to the data and become collaborators in a reflexive process with the evidence of their own practice in their own social world, with the insight and understandings of the researcher, and with their own self-reflection as a form of self-critique and ideology critique.

The openly ideological nature of critical inquiry means that a critical ethnography of clinical nursing practice is research in and for nursing and not just about it (Carr and Kemmis 1983). This means that not only socially constituted nursing hierarchies need to be examined but the hierarchies of the research process itself. Research that claims an emancipatory intent needs to be careful that it is not perpetuating the oppression of the research participants by disempowering them in the research process. Reifying the theoretical constructions of the researcher over the values and understandings held by practitioners endorses the theory/practice gap. Emancipatory researchers need to engage in a dialogue of collaborative reflection, which poses questions about actions and subjects those actions to systematic scrutiny and debate as a basis for changed understandings and changed actions.

In this ethnography I compiled comprehensive descriptive accounts of the clinical practice of four nurses giving them back the research accounts for ongoing analysis and critique. This process of continually sharing the research data, and my emerging theoretical constructions, with the nurses required them to engage in collaborative reflection and theory development. The process of problematising the everyday taken-for-granted activities of nurses and the contexts in which these actions were embedded served to nurture a process of consciousness-raising of the nurses engaged in the study at the same time as it worked to inform and transform problems and perspectives about clinical nursing formerly held by the researcher. These changed understandings formed the basis of changed actions.

The process of problematising clinical nursing practice is not without its problems in relation to language use and interpretation. The development of reciprocity in collaborative dialogue is not a neutral exercise because the way in which the dialogue is formed and used depends greatly upon the agreed upon worldview of the researcher and research participants. Rational dialogue is not an objective entity but is enacted by historical and embodied human beings who are as capable of engaging in rationally constructed disagreements about knowledge and action as in rationally constructed agreements. Through the reflexive process of collaborative discourse contradictions in theories, values, and actions are identified.

The Significance of the Study

> It is our belief that the "real" expertise of clinicians lies in their ability to learn to manage the complexities and multiplicities of every here and now situation which they encounter...Clinical nurses...recognize that effective practice requires skill in making numerous, complex judgements which effect idiosyncratic practices which appropriately are situation specific...Clinical experts have gained their everyday understandings from their engagement in and lived experiences of nursing. (Cox and Moss 1988:4)

Nurses are beginning to acknowledge the complexity of nursing knowledge. An International Nursing Conference in December 1988 took as the conference theme the title "Professional Promiscuity" in acknowledgement of the disparate, disordered complexity of elements that make up the sociocultural world of nursing practice. Cox and Moss (1988) have argued that promiscuous knowledge is reflected in the chaos of clinical nursing practice and that an acceptance of this chaotic nature brings with it the challenge to develop new ways of understanding the nature of nursing practice and the knowledge base of expert practitioners. They suggest that contemporary nursing literature represents clinical practice as based on principles and rules, which are orderly, logical, and systematic. According to Cox and Moss this orderliness can only be discerned in the routines in which nurses engage, and these routines themselves are practiced within a simultaneous multiplicity of events. Schön (1987) likens professional practice to a varied topography consisting of high, hard ground overlooking a swamp. The high, hard ground consists of the resolution of manageable problems through the application of research-based theory and technique. Schön claims that these manageable problems that occupy the hard high ground, while often of great technical interest, tend to be relatively unimportant either to the individual or to society.

The high hard ground is familiar to nursing scholars. It is also the area that clinicians often regard as irrelevant to the real task of nursing. For clinical nurses the contextual realities—the leaking tube, the atypical patient, the hysterical relative, the demanding doctor, the unrealistic roster, the continual interruptions, the malfunctioning technology, the bureaucratic bun-gle, and the ethical quandary—combine to represent the swampy lowlands of practice. According to Schön this swampy lowland consists of messy, confusing problems that not only defy technical solution but are those problems of greatest concern to humanity. The challenge is for the practitioner to move from the safety of easily resolved but relatively unimportant problems and to take the risk of pursuing answers to the problems that are important for them.

Lather (1985:8) reminds us that "we are both shaped by and shapers of our world." She argues for a process of research on practice that enables practitioners to empower themselves to change their understandings, their actions, and the situation in the practice setting. She argues that our choice of research paradigms reflect our beliefs about the world we live in and want to live in. Lather suggests that we need research designs that allow us to reflect on how our value commitments insert themselves into our empirical work. Our own frameworks of understanding need to be critically examined as we look for the tensions and contradictions they might entail

> ...the search is for theory which grows out of context embedded data, not in a way that rejects a priori theory, but in a way that keeps it from distorting the logic of evidence. Theory is too often used to protect us from the awesome complexity of the world. (Lather 1985:25)

To experience the awesome complexity of clinical nursing practice is to spend time in the swamp; to lay aside preconceived expectations and unexamined habits; to reject mythical thinking and easy solutions to well-known questions. Nurses need to put their role as a nurse, their nursing actions, and the clinical setting in which they practice under close scrutiny as a basis for critical analysis and reflection.The reflection process is demanding. It is easier to search for the high hard ground of problem-solving exercises. The way through the swamp, the way of reflection, requires an examination of the reality as it is. This pathway does not contain known problems waiting to be solved. Instead it poses dilemmas with more than one equally acceptable option; options that are consistent with different value stances and ways of understanding the world of clinical practice. Reflection does not begin with a search for answers but with a search for questions (Freire 1972).

The reflective process begins with a reconstruction of experience, which is recorded for analysis. This analytical process not only uncovers the personal and nursing issues and meanings at work in the situation, but uncovers the historical and social factors that have shaped both the nurse and the clinical setting. This analysis forms the basis of a problem-setting exercise where problems are posed to enable the nurse to question the tacit ways of knowing and practicing nursing. This confrontation of the experience, and of the meanings and assumptions which surround it, can form a foundation upon which to make choices about future actions based on chosen value stances and new ways of thinking about, and understanding, nursing practice.

Critical reflection on clinical nursing practice has been ignored for a long time. Nurse educators have continued to prepare nursing students in curricula processes that support and develop technical and, more recently, practical knowledge. A concern for the patient as the focus of nursing practice has led many educators to develop curricula based on positivist psychological research. This curricula is dominated by a desire to reduce human behavior to categories for description, classification, and theory building. This reductionist approach endeavors to develop theory to be applied by practitioners, while ignoring the contextual, idiosyncratic realities of nursing practice. Perry and Moss (1988) contend that nursing needs to reject the utilitarian concept of knowledge and explore the dialectical relationship between theory and practice. They argue for the introduction of transformative curriculum processes based on critical self-reflection and rational debate. However, to engage in education through a transformative curriculum is to assume that the educator has a knowledge of clinical nursing practice that is enlightened, empowering, and emancipatory. This kind of knowledge has not been documented in Australia, and it appears that this area of research has also been neglected overseas. Nurse educators interested in pursuing a critical approach have focused on curricula development in order to develop an emancipated nurse (Perry 1985a; Perry and Moss 1988; Cox and Moss 1988; Yuen 1987).

My experience would suggest that the more generalized critical analysis possible in a critical ethnography is a useful and possibly necessary methodology. The field of nursing has used methods, such as action research, in authoritarian and nonliberating ways by not questioning the power/knowledge basis upon which nursing is structured before engaging in actions designed to bring about local, context-specific change.

I would suggest that this study is significant because it endorses the view that clinical nurses can pursue empowering knowledge and engage in emancipatory action. It focuses on the neglected area of clinical practice as a basis for a collaborative critical inquiry into nursing. It is premised on the belief that a critical examination of nursing practice is long overdue and is a necessary basis for a transformative curriculum.

Limitations of the Study

The limitations of this study pertain to its context of clinical nursing practice, the administrative practices surrounding clinical nurses, and the research methodology employed.

The study was pursued in the dynamic environment of clinical nursing practice, which, like most large structured bureaucracies, does not represent an integrated whole with power relations operating in clearly identifiable configurations. Rather, it has developed as a result of a multiplicity of unrelated decisions, actions, interrelations, emergencies, and unintended consequences. This multifaceted meshing of power relations worked at times to support the research, but often it worked to limit and shape the research. Access to the research site was well supported by senior nursing staff. However, other factors, such as nursing mobility throughout the hospital, last-minute changes to shifts, the needs of other individuals within the hospital, and other difficulties related to continually negotiating privacy and confidentiality with an everchanging group of patients and co-workers, meant that the data collected in an ethnography based on following around specific nurses is more individual and context-specific than the data collected from a stable unit such as a ward.

The methodology enabled the researcher to collect large amounts of data, which was highly specific to nurses in a large acute hospital, and as such it highlighted issues and generated questions for more structured and specific research into clinical nursing practice. Nurses used in the case studies were all very experienced nurses who were fully employed in nursing and intended to continue in the field. They were all female and white Australians. Although the hospital employs nurses from

European and Asian ethnic background, there were none
working in the areas that I had access to. This part of Melbourne has very few blacks, and I saw no black staff or
patients throughout the nine-month period of the study. The
data is, therefore, contextual and specific to these kind of
nurses in Victoria and not necessarily generalizable to, or representative of, neophyte nurses, part-time nurses, nurses from
places with different cultural, social, and/or educational
preparation or nurses in nonacute settings. Therefore,
although the major issues remain the same, the focus and
specifics could be very varied. The research problem, choice of
focus, theoretical basis, and methodology represent the knowledge, skills, and interests of the researcher and the nurses in
the case study and was therefore limited by the researcher, the
participants, and the research process.

Any research design that claims to be openly ideological
and emancipatory in intent using reflection and critical discourse requires examination. A critical ethnography is conducted by an "outsider," the researcher as participant observer,
who collaborates with the "insider," the research participants,
to engage in an in-depth case study with a deliberate agenda
directed towards emancipatory knowledge and action. This
research was limited to recording and analyzing the observable
nursing actions and the outwardly manifested interactions as
a basis for later discussion with the nurses. The researcher,
who is not a nurse, was reliant on the critical interpretations
jointly agreed upon by the nurses and herself. This differed
from those other critical research methods, such as action
research, where the researcher is also the practitioner putting
her own practices under scrutiny. However, the power/knowl-
edge and emancipatory focus required the researcher to critique both her role and actions as researcher in order to reveal
the contradictions and dilemmas faced by researchers during
the act of researching and theorizing.

The purpose of the research can govern aspects of the
research such as the content, shape, length, complexity, and
form of reporting. This research was being conducted within a
particular time frame to meet the requirements of a doctor of
philosophy degree. The research was designed to be emancipatory in intent, design, and conduct. It was initially intended
that the research would be entirely collaborative and that the
research participants would engage in coauthorship of sections

of the final report. This was a naive assumption, which demonstrated the difference in understandings held by myself, other academics, and the nurses themselves concerning the possibilities and the realities of collaborative research for a higher degree. The intention to engage nurses in sharing the writing task with me about issues in nursing practice demonstrated my naiveté in understanding the oral culture of nursing and the structured differences between this and the academic culture based on "publish or perish." It was not sufficient to encourage nurses to write about nursing issues, or to journal their nursing practices, because they saw no more reason to change from their oral culture and accommodate me than they did with the administrative injunctions to write up nursing care plans. The nurses engaged in the same passive resistance with me as they did in their workplace, and this passive resistance helped me to identify a telling contradiction in my own research practice. In attempting to develop collaboration based on coauthorship, I was imposing a collaborative style that disempowered these nurses, who were highly articulate within their oral culture but felt disempowered when required to document their own understandings. The nurses were always cooperative in their own ways, and it was only as I reflected in my journal upon the intentions of the research design that I recognized that I was intending to use my power/knowledge to bring about a change in their mode of expression in order to fit in with my research design. Through negotiation I was able to redesign the research to take account of the strengths of the oral character of nursing culture.

This put the onus for transcribing tapes, writing notes, and forming or systematizing arguments back onto me. I decided this also was appropriate because I was the one who would benefit from the award of a Ph.D. if the research was satisfactory. I shelved my cherished dream of coauthorship, which would have given the nurses an opportunity to publicly argue their views. I reflected that the Ph.D. would not be awarded to me unless I could demonstrate my capacity to research and theorize at a level that would not be expected of clinical nurses without undergraduate degrees, and yet I was committed to the view that these nurses knew best how to theorize about their clinical nursing practice. This commitment was validated by the capacity of the nurses to respond orally to my challenges, to theorize in a sophisticated manner concerning the historical constructions and contradictions in clinical practice, and to enable me to learn from their cultural perspectives in ways that changed my understandings and the theoretical shape of the research.

The research was limited by a time frame that was deemed appropriate for the researcher's question and the needs of the nurses. The research was also conducted within a particular context within a large typical general hospital in Melbourne, Australia, during 1987. This was a time when many nurses were beginning to question nursing practices as a result of the 1986 nurses' strike and the subsequent inquiry into professional issues in nursing in Victoria. The research design enabled nurses to ask and pursue their own questions as well as collaborate with the questions raised by the researcher. The data was initially shaped by the actions of the nurses and by their comments and taped discussions. In these settings the nurses developed themes and issues of interest to them, and I raised those themes and issues that I was identifying in the data. However, the extent to which I had to organize and, therefore, select the focus of the research was a dilemma, particularly when individual nurses had other interests, such as nursing stress or the development of appropriate nursing care for geriatric patients, which also could be developed from the data but which needed a much more in-depth treatment than was possible within the research. I recognized my own role in the collaborative meaning-making process as the interpreter of the theorizing process and of the theoretical constructions and implications that were emerging from the data. My reflections upon the data and upon the nurses' reflections shaped the theoretical arguments to which they responsed and engaged in further reflection.

A dilemma is faced by the ethnographic researcher regarding the amount of data that is collected through participant observation that needs to be focused and refined. The power/knowledge and subsequent nurturance/knowledge focus of the research could have been pursued through the data in many other ways. The seemingly disparate data was organized and constructed in particular ways that followed our research interests.

A further dilemma related to the impact on the research process of the evolving theory, which I was generating. There was an emergent recognition of a dialectical relationship in which the nurturance/knowledge aspect challenged the power/knowledge construction of the research and challenged the way in which the research was being conducted. I realized that I could not only reflect on my own actions as researcher in the light of power/knowledge, but I also needed to examine them through the challenges of this nurturance/knowledge, perspective. Only when I really begin to recognize the nurturance/ knowledge theory at work was I able to understand that I could change the conduct of the research to value the oral culture of nursing and use it in the research. This was an empowering experience for me. The power/knowledge focus left nurses disempowered through their lack of engagement in written documentation, but the nurturance/knowledge focus demonstrated the negativity of power/knowledge and the positive capacity for nurses to develop critique and contestation. The examination of the unspoken values underpinning clinical practice highlighted the rationales for action, which remained obscure within the power/knowledge grid and encouraged me to examine my unspoken valuing of the written code of academic culture over oral nursing culture. Reflection on these dilemmas helped further the research process, my own understandings of my theoretical biases, and the possibilities inherent in new questions and reconstructions of theory.

The processes of collaboration and negotiation themselves posed dilemmas for me because I had underestimated the difficulty of getting nurses together to discuss issues from their practice. Research that is conducted using students from university courses or from an employment situation where the researcher has an official status is much more manageable because the participants are required to participate through official or unofficial sanctions and power relationships. My only previous experiences of researching with independent volunteers was with social workers who were used to developing and participating in group work. They were predisposed to group work through their social work education and their participation in therapy groups and feminist groups. I soon discovered that the structuring of nursing practice and the demands of shift work meant that nurses generally have limited opportunities to participate in groups for sharing and collaborative reflection for either personal or professional reasons. My group work expectations were a product of my own middle-class personal and professional history, and this realization challenged me to justify the necessity of the group work focus for the research. Although I still believe that the research would have been more effective had I acted as a facilitator and recorder of change processes during group work, I also recognized that group work would need to be a decision entered into freely by the research participants. These research participants were already giving generously of their limited free time and they scattered to different hospitals during the research; therefore, it was obviously not feasible. Nevertheless, collaborative group work is something I would consider carefully and attempt to negotiate into future research designs.

The questions of *when, where,* and *how* to end the research posed a further dilemma. I was keen to pursue more and more questions and found it difficult in this kind of interactive study to terminate the research. Essentially I opened up a number of areas to be pursued by myself and others. The interactive approach meant that I developed satisfying relationships with the nurses concerned. It was difficult to break off these stimulating discussions particularly when we had engaged in sharing experiences and knowledge in depth. I found that I was in the same situation as Oakley (1981) when she engaged in a reciprocity of sharing in her interviews with women, which led to the development of a few real friendships. McRobbie (1982) in her comments on Oakley's situation suggests that it was a measure of the powerlessness of these women that they did collaborate and form relationships with a caring, articulate researcher who was interested in them and in their opinions. I think that some of the nurses have continued to initiate contact with me because they do enjoy talking about nursing with someone who is interested in learning about nursing from them and who is prepared to take their views seriously as a basis for critique and reconstruction. If this process demonstrated the powerlessness of nurses, it also demonstrated the powerlessness of this isolated researcher pursing doctoral studies who experienced the nurturance/knowledge construct at work when the nurses also took her views seriously and helped her make sense of their world of clinical nursing. I believe this demonstrates the nurses' commitment to nurturance/knowledge because the interactive process enabled us to provide each other with mutual respect, support, and knowledge through the process of critique and reconstruction.

The process of engaging in this research was enlightening,

empowering, and emancipatory for me as researcher. *Enlightenment* came through the development of my knowledge of clinical nurses, their working situation and the limitations of the power/knowledge theoretical framework with which I had chosen to examine clinical nursing practice. The processes of observation, critique, and collaborative meaning making enabled me to identify many theoretical constructs, such as accommodation and resistance at work, and through analysis I was able to develop new theoretical insights into nursing practice.

These insights were *empowering*, because they enabled me to move beyond the realm of recognizing and using methodological techniques and theory devised by others, into the realm of creating empowering collaborative research practices and theory development informed by the nurses and with which they experienced face validity. It was the initial "yes, but" responses of the interactive face validity process that facilitated the development of new theory and the affirming "yes, that's right" response. Interactive collaboration took away the power to reconstruct a lone view of reality, empowering participants and researcher through the process of contestation and critique.

Emancipation is demonstrated through action. An ethnography does not facilitate action for its research participants in the manner of more action-oriented methodologies such as action research. However, the nurses did respond to our collaborative critiques by actions designed to change the situation. Some actions were emancipatory, but many reflected the dominance of the technical model in nursing practice when nurses who had arrived at strategic action plans through collaborative analysis then attempted to impose them hierarchically rather than facilitate a collaborative process for contestation and negotiation among nursing colleagues. Nonviolent emancipatory change takes a commitment to ideology critique and negotiated collaborative strategies for change and takes time. This process involves self-reflection to disclose the historical construction, values, ethics, and taken-for-grantedness of habitual practices while accounting for the embodied and embedded character of social actors and the limits to freedom, rationality, and happiness, which constrain and shape their world of practice. This study was just a beginning.

2

❦

Situating the Journey

This research journey was conducted at a specific historio-political junction in nursing in Australia. Therefore, an examination of the sociocultural context within which the specific research context was located is important as is the identification of the issues that were perculating in the nursing community in Australia at this time.

Clinical Nursing Practice: Crisis in Context

Fay (1987) argues that the practical intent of critical social science is only appropriate when a social group is in crisis and so is unable to continue to function as it had in the past. He differentiates between a social crisis and social conflict by suggesting that within a state of crisis there are no options for continuance and that change of some kind is inevitable. By contrast, social conflict may be represented by a high level of discontent within the structure of the social group, but this discontent is managed through social mechanisms that maintain an equilibrium, which tolerates a level of conflict.

This study of clinical nursing practice was conducted at a time when Victorian nursing had moved beyond the previously stable situation of conflict, which was maintained and managed by accommodating strategies that recreated the existing power relationships. The data collection stage of the study coincided with the aftermath of the most obvious manifestation of the crisis situation in nursing in Victoria—the historic 1986

Royal Australian Nursing Federation (RANF) nurses' strike. Although an in-depth analysis of the mechanics of the strike is inappropriate in the context of this study, the strike itself is important because it had the effect of politicizing nurses and nursing issues that had previously been confined to the area of academic debate.

Crisis in the Making

According to Willis (1983) the Victorian healthcare system reflects the class and gender relations of the wider society. He contends that class interests are reflected directly and ideologically within the social organization of healthcare. The direct effect of these class interests are demonstrated through relations of domination and subordination. Willis, following Weber, argues that these class-based relations of domination are power relations. These are distinct from authority relations, which also enact domination and subordination but are not based on class. Burbules (1986) suggests that the authority of doctors is not only supported by their special knowledge but also with institutional arrangements, which have little to do with authority and much to do with the maintenance of class-based privilege.

The ideological component of class is evident in the complex and contradictory theories and practices that result in differentiation in the health division of labor. This differentiation needs to be viewed in the context of the economic and political relations of the state. The labeling and management of illness through state-legitimated and -financed forms of treatment supports the maintenance of a healthcare system that is compatible with dominant class interests. This state patronage occurs through the regulation and funding arrangements, by the Health Department, of a hierarchical healthcare system, which enables the class structure of the community to be reproduced in the dominance of the medical profession over other healthcare providers with concomitant access to education, resources, and privilege. The state has not only legalized medical dominance but legally limits the roles, relationships, and access to resources of the other members of the healthcare team such as nurses. These class-instituted and -supported relationships of dominance and subordination at a macro level of healthcare are reflected on a micro level in the structuring of relationships of power and dominance between doctors and nurses working together in healthcare settings. Medical hegemony is maintained by class interests in the form of elite education, legal sanctions, political, economic, social, and cultural practices.

Interrelating with and pervading class relations in the social construction of healthcare in Victoria are gender relations. Gender relations represent the ways in which masculinity and femininity are socially constructed (Game 1983). These gender relations are evident in all spheres of society, but in the healthcare system the sexual division of labor is evident in the development of dominance and subordination in the structuring of occupational roles. In this context nursing is recognized as a female-dominated profession, which is subjugated to the male-dominated medical profession. These constructions of class and gender relations will be developed further in later chapters. However, it is important to recognize that they form the basis upon which an understanding of the crisis in nursing is expressed in the issues and the actions of the strike.

The path that led to this particular industrial situation is grounded in nursing history formed by class and gender relations, but it is useful to identify particular benchmarks in its progress. In 1977 the Victorian government introduced staff ratios and staff ceilings in all government-funded hospitals. These staff ceilings initially caused some unrest but became increasingly unrealistic as the nursing role developed to encompass more medical and technical procedures. Alarmed at the heavy staff losses incurred as dissatisfied nurses left the public hospital system, the unions developed strategies of protest such as "work-to-rule." This was followed by the designation of "nonnursing duties" as some tasks were redefined as more appropriate for ancillary staff than registered nurses. This action and the following negotiations between hospitals, government, and unions culminated in the introduction of ward clerks and nursing assistants. Despite these initiatives, increasing numbers of nurses continued to vote with their feet and either leave nursing altogether or move into nonclinical roles in nurse education, administration, or research.

In 1985 the Health Department and the RANF began formal discussions aimed at developing a career structure and appropriate pay rates to reverse the exodus of clinical nurses from nursing practice. In June 1986 the State Industrial Relations Commission handed down a decision on a new wages and career structure for nurses. The decision was not acceptable to the members of the RANF because of a number of anomalies, one of the most serious being the apparent demotion of some senior staff with corresponding wage decreases as a result of the restructuring of the clinical roles. The union presented a log of twenty claims to the commission for conciliation. The commission claimed that conciliation was not possible and threatened to begin arbitration procedures. The union took action and called out its members on a series of isolated rolling strikes.The nonresolution of the log of claims by negotiation led to an escalation of the rolling strikes.

On Friday 31 October 1986 Victorian nurses began the first statewide strike of clinical nurses. The strike lasted for fifty days and became a watershed in the history of clinical nursing practice in Victoria. By their action nurses joined a growing list of occupations whose members were considered "essential services" but who nevertheless had lost patience with the arbitration process and gone on strike. Notably, the earliest Australian "essential service" unions to strike were the male-dominated unions such as miners and transport workers who held crippling national and statewide strikes from 1938 (Connell 1977). Female-dominated occupations such as primary education and welfare eventually followed suit and instituted strike action to achieve their union claims. Nursing, which is female-dominated but historically subjugated to the male-dominated medical profession, had neither the unity within its own numbers nor the commitment to an improvement in the conditions for all nurses to take strike action until 1986. Therefore, the strike represented the first major collective response to inequities and oppression of nurses in clinical nursing practice although, as previously stated, individual nurses had responded by leaving nursing in ever-increasing numbers. The collective action represented by the strike owed much to the effects of the changed awareness of roles, rights, and responsibilities of women in the general community. This awareness enabled nurses to decide that they did not have to take responsibility for the inequities in the health system despite the emotionally charged community accusations that strike action had led to deaths in the community. Nurses answered this charge with the countercharge that people had been dying unnecessarily for some time in Victoria as a result of a shortage of nurses, which constantly put pressure on existing staff and put patients at risk.

The strong gender base of nursing meant that not only did they receive criticism from the public and the male-dominated class interests of government, hospital administration, and medicine, but they did not receive the solidarity which is traditionally received from other trade unions. Mark Davis (1986), chief industrial reporter for *The Age* newspaper, contends that this occurred because the Australian industrial relations system is male-dominated and characterized by "macho posturings." He argued that the inclusion of nursing union leaders into this domain caused considerable confusion. The nurses refused to follow the traditional unwritten rules and procedures of this macho industrial relations game and so became the target of sexual politics—innuendo, sexist remarks, patronizing tactics, slurs upon personal lifestyle, and hunts to try to locate the "strongmen" behind the female nursing leaders (Davis 1986).

Although this industrial experience was new to nursing, the issue of sexual politics is not. The strike enabled many middle-class and working-class women to identify their oppression as nurses and as women in relation to the upper-class male oppressors of government, health administration, and medicine. This relationship between class and gender identification as represented in the issues of the strike were identified daily by nurses writing to the press in defense of their industrial action. Ruth Smith, RN, (1986) wrote

Nursing has traditionally been a female profession, and thus has suffered the many inequalities faced by women in the workforce at large...We have suffered lack of power in our healthcare institutions, little say in decision-making processes that affect our work environment, a heavy workload with few means to control it, a handmaiden/ ministering angel image, low professional status (particularly compared to doctors), and our own generally passive, non-assertive nature...it is not just money and career structure that is at stake here, we are trying to shrug off a whole tradition of submission and oppression. What the community is witnessing is our revolution—not just industrially, but in our thinking. We, as women, and as nurses (apologies to all the male nurses), are standing up and declaring our rights.

The relationship of the strike to the powerlessness that nurses have felt indicates a growing awareness of the ways in which they have been implicated in the processes of their own oppression and in the oppression of others (Fay 1977). Infante (1985) describes the consequences of this oppression of clinical nurses as low status, poor image, male domination, poor economic rewards, and generally inadequate educational facilities. Menzies-Lyth (1986) argues that nurses experience their powerlessness as alienation, depersonalization, and devaluation. She believes that nurses are feeling diminished and frustrated, and she contends that these emotional conditions can lead to despair. Coping with despair leads nurses to fragment the core problems into seemingly manageable practical problems as a defense about their anxiety at facing something of such magnitude. These fragmented practical problems are then projected onto ambients (fringe benefits) and a feeling that something needs to be done by unknown others to rectify their situation. Anger then can be expressed at unknown authority figures for not dealing with the fragments of the problem. Strike action may improve the ambients through changes in fringe benefits but will increase the stress and guilt carried by nurses intensifying the core problems that are not being addressed by the demands for improved work conditions.

Fay (1977) argues that the way to free people from the causes of their oppression is through the revelation of the existence and the precise nature of these causes. This revelation and identification robs the causal mechanisms of their power. Nurses are just beginning to feel that they have some power and want to retain that situation.

> Nurses cannot return to work without achieving something positive. After many years of feeling powerless, we have found a new strength through united action and enormous personal struggle. The psychological effect of being proven still powerless would be devastating to nursing morale and the future healthcare of Victorians. (Mann 1986)

Freire (1981) argues that when emotion, rather than critical reflection, is the basis for radical action, the understanding of power can be distorted in mythical and illogical ways. He suggests that when action is based on emotions, people can become objects, while believing themselves to be subjects and to be free. He describes the emotional power of the transition from oppression to freedom as occurring when the oppressed understand the extent of their oppression, and the extent to which the oppressors hold them in contempt, and tend to react aggressively. This provokes fear in the oppressors, of a threat to the legitimacy of their power, leading to measures to silence and domesticate the oppressed. This emergence of an ill-prepared, emotional group of reactive people who are oppressed can leave them a ready target for irrational choices and behavior.

Although many nurses experienced some heady moments of freedom and collegiality during the strike, these were balanced by intense feelings of guilt, confusion, anger, frustration, and increasing division and dissension between nurses and nurses, nurses and other hospital employees, and nurses and the general public. Since the strike ended nurses have generally merged back into their same roles in health settings, financially richer and more politicized concerning nursing issues but without yet achieving freedom from the oppressive elements of their situation—evidence of the ability of the dominant culture to silence and domesticate opposition.

I contend that Bullough's (1984) concern with the importance of an understanding of role in resistance is useful for nursing. Much of the confusion of the strike emanated from disagreements as to the role of nurses. Nurses need to examine Bullough's challenge to teachers and recognize that roles have histories and are formed interactively. Therefore, the challenge is one of

> defining role, of reshaping it, and of building supportive institutional structures and shared understandings...As role becomes less taken-for-granted, less ideologically embedded...resistance becomes those acts that press up against role boundaries. (Bullough 1984:96)

I began by suggesting that the strike was a watershed for nurses. It enabled many nurses to be exposed to ideas and attitudes that were radical and critical of medical and nursing culture, and of the social hegemony that supports them. For most nurses the strike could be categorized more as a spontaneous reaction from an oppressed group rather than a predetermined position based on rational thinking and dialogue. This meant that powerful societal constraints—government, media, doctors, public opinion—were able to keep the group divided, both within its own ranks and on the key issues involved. Despite these pressures the strike mobilized and radicalized nurses. They received pay rises and some changes in nursing conditions, but more importantly they began to talk and think about clinical nursing and ways in which to bring about transformation and emancipation.

A Response to the Crisis:
The Study on Professional Issues in Nursing

The strike had begun with industrial concerns about wages and conditions, but when some concessions and consensus had been won on these issues it became apparent that the striking nurses had widened their agenda and were including other issues. These issues were being identified as the core issues of which the ambients of wages and conditions were symptomatic. In response to this emergence of issues that were potentially much more challenging to the hegemony of the healthcare system, the Victorian government commissioned a committee to address the issues raised during the strike and to prepare a report with recommendations for future action. In this manner the so-called Marles Report, named after Fay Marles, the chair of the committee, joined the plethora of reports on nursing in Victoria.

The terms of reference of the report reflect the key areas identified by representatives of the state Health Department, nursing educators, and RANF representatives. These issues mirrored those identified by nurses and journalists during the extensive media coverage of the strike. They highlight the changing role of nurses and the nature of nursing; the relationships with other healthcare providers; the effects of the advances in medical science and technology; the implications of the changing nature of nursing education; and the issues regarding the female nature of nursing at a time when the changing role of women in Western society has become widely accepted. It was not within the scope of the report to locate these issues theoretically within the debates of nursing or in relation to nursing literature. The evidence considered by the study was provided by a wide spectrum of nurses representing divergent experience, education, skills, interests, and degree of engagement in clinical practice. Submissions were also received from other groups and individuals with vested interest in the outcomes of the report such as health administrators, educators, doctors, and members of paramedical specialities. The evidence presented was informed by prior experience, by nursing, medical, and community attitudes, and through debate prior to and during the strike. Much of the debate rightly identifies the cultural, historical, social, and political forces that have shaped the development of these issues. However, many of the excursions into nursing history and culture have formulated deterministic explanations of the roles of nurses and their relationships to the state, other healthcare professions, healthcare administrators, ethical practices, and to the female nature of nursing. These explanations locate the issues within the constraints of the existing social organization of healthcare rather than challenging the taken-for-grantedness of the construction of nursing knowledge and practice.

The committee demonstrated an awareness of the limitations of reports and recommendations to facilitate change in nursing practice in its opening remarks.

Over the last decade there has been much debate and several inquiries into aspects of nursing in Australia. It is the sense of the profession that this has resulted in no appreciable change. (Marles 1988:1)

The report then goes on to quote two submissions that highlighted the scepticism and concerns felt by nurses towards studies and reports, which are authorized by successive governments whenever there is severe industrial disruption. They claimed that these reports reiterate the same issues, that recommendations are always ignored and that nurses believe that no previous nursing inquiry had led to tangible action. The committee identified the three objectives of the study as

(i) to achieve a better understanding of the professional issues in nursing; (ii) to identify policies and practices that needed to be introduced or changed for the greater effectiveness of nursing; and (iii) to make recommendations on ways to achieve the desired change (page 3).

This orientation supports the notion that changes in nursing practice will be developed hierarchically by government action and intervention rather than by changes in knowledge and practice by clinical practitioners themselves. In fairness to the members of the committee, they had little choice to develop anything other than functional recommendations directed to different powerful groups interested in, and responsible for, the structures within which nursing is practiced. These recommendations will enable Health authorities to provide some limited concessions and adjustments to the system while re-creating and maintaining their own hegemonic control.

The re-creation of hegemony through the process of responding to the ambients rather than the core problems is demonstrated in the recommendations relating to the issues of gender relations within the healthcare system. Despite raising and clarifying some important and telling arguments for oppression by gender in nursing, the committee limited themselves to recommending that hospital management explore options for part-time job-sharing roster patterns, for self-rostering and for the use of computerized nurse allocation systems. While being useful, these recommendations are essentially institutional and structural changes that can be operationalized without disturbing the power relations of domination and subordination by gender within hospitals. The only other relevant recommendation was concerned with doctor-nurse relationships and suggested that problems in this area would be solved through better understanding of each other's priorities and processes, something that the report suggested "should not, in the long term, be unduly difficult" if educational institutions preparing medical and nursing students investigate the possibility of some interdisciplinary teaching (Marles 1988:260, 262). This response ignores the historical problems of medical staff teaching in nursing courses, which has been a contributing factor in the subordination of nursing. It is also naive concerning the hegemony of medical dominance when it assumes that nurse participation in medical education could be more than tokenism. This naiveté ignores the structures of resistance to nursing interventions in the acculturation process of educating doctors to act as a member of the dominant medical elite class.

It appears unlikely that this report as a product will have any significant influence on the problems facing clinical nursing practice. Certainly many of the recommendations will be ignored, many will be reinterpreted by government officials, and the irrelevance of enquiries of this kind to the core issues under discussion will be reinforced yet again. However, the decision taken by the committee members to actively encourage nurses to talk and write about nursing issues facilitated a process of analysis and reflection that reinforced the politicizing process of the strike. The large number of contributors to this report demonstrates that clinical nurses are beginning a process by which they could begin to develop a dialogue of protest with potential for transformative action.

This then is the context in which the data collection stage of observing and engaging with nurses in an analysis of their practice occurred. The main issues raised during the strike and within the report will now be examined in further detail drawing upon the literature, which has been informing the shaping and formulation of these issues from the context of clinical practice.

3

❦

The Doctor Knows Best

Just as in the world-wide provision of health-care women
are more important than men, so nurses are quite indis-
putedly more important than doctors.

(Oakley 1986:181)

With these provocative words Ann Oakley begins her
chapter entitled "On the importance of being a Nurse" in
Telling the Truth about Jerusalem (1986). Oakley acknowledges
that this is not the dominant view of public opinion and that it
is a view she has only come to adopt after fifteen years of
blindness, paradoxically within her career as a medical sociolo-
gist, to the contribution made by nurses to healthcare. However, her view of the relative importance of nursing and medicine
is not a view subscribed to by the general community, by
medicine, and indeed by many nurses. What is the meaning
for the community of a hierarchical view of healthcare
providers that places medical knowledge at the apex of the
pyramid? How does this relegation of nursing to a subservient
position within the healthcare hierarchy affect the healthcare
received by the community? These questions have their concerns in the structured dominance of medicine and its implications for nursing knowledge and nursing care.

Medical Dominance and the Implications for Nursing

Doctors and nurses are key players in the provision of public
healthcare, and so medical dominance has important implica-

tions not only for the nursing profession but for the healthcare of the wider community. The medical profession has achieved a virtually unchallenged professional status, which, with the support of state legal protection, has enabled them to dominate and control the development of nursing. This dominance has meant that doctors have been implicated in the oppression of nurses and that nurses have been implicated in their own oppression when some nurse leaders have identified with the doctors and worked to "police" the oppression of their peers.

The Medical Profession

The claim that medicine is a profession has long gone unchallenged. Medicine not only carries the legacy of its historical position as a profession, along with law and the church, but, unlike them, the medical profession has in modern times been allied with the gods of science and technology. Friedson (1970) describes the characteristics of a profession as

> ...an occupation which has assumed a dominant position in a division of labor, so that it gains control over the determination of the substance of its own work...it claims to be the most reliable authority on the nature of the reality it deals with...(it) changes the definition and shape of the problems as experienced by the layman. The layman's problem is re-created as it is managed—a new social reality is created by...the autonomous position of the profession in society. (p.xvii)

Larson (1977) develops this further with an emphasis on the status seeking and collective upward mobility of emerging professions; their use of control not only in relation to individuals and other occupational groups but of economic markets; and the ideological nature of their claim to autonomy. This ability to dominate other occupational groups by providing the normative view of reality has enabled medicine to be seen as "a prototype upon which occupations seeking a privileged status today are modelling their aspirations" (Friedson 1970). Medicine has developed a state-sanctioned, legally supported monopoly over healthcare. This is practiced in a variety of ways, the most obvious being the legalized medical monopoly over prescriptions for drugs, over the use of sophisticated technological interventions in healthcare practice and over the work of other health professionals, either by referral to therapists and specialists or by direct control as in the case of nurses. This medical monopoly provides high economic rewards and access to political influence—an influence that enables medicine to discourage competitors such as alternate health practitioners and to subordinate others under its sphere of influence thereby re-creating and redefining the sociocultural construction of health issues and healthcare (Willis 1983).

The legitimation of medicine is a process by which medicine operates as an institution of social control reproducing the dominant ideology of healthcare in a hegemonic relationship with the state. This social control is effected in two main ways. According to Ehrenreich (1978), disciplinary control enables doctors to function both implicitly and explicitly to discourage the entry of particular individuals into a sick role, which would prevent attendance at work or in family responsibilities. This control supports the expansion of medicine by designating particular sick roles as appropriate, and so develops the professional management of various aspects of the lives of people who have been designated "sick" or as needing medical help, even when they are well, through the medicalization of areas such as prevention, contraception, or marital difficulties. Legitimation of these forms of social control is based on an acceptance that medicine operates from a basis of "superior" knowledge to that which forms the basis of other health disciplines. This hierarchical ordering of knowledge affords superiority to knowledge produced by the natural sciences and used in the practice of medicine and medical technology while denigrating practical knowledge that forms the basis of much of the distinct knowledge of paramedical disciplines and nursing. This alignment of medicine with the knowledge of the natural sciences denies the ideological component of medicine, which has its material reality in clinical practices. This ideological knowledge contains the ethical, social, cultural, and artistic components of medical knowledge and practice. Therefore, although scientific and ideological knowledge are treated as analytically distinct, they fuse in medicine in clinical practice.

The hegemonic hierarchical ordering of claims to ownership of legitimate knowledge not only supports the dominance of medicine but has been used historically as a mechanism to deskill other health disciplines. The widespread utilization of forceps by male doctors in childbirth during the seventeenth and eighteenth centuries began a process of deskilling female midwives (Ehrenreich 1973). Political strategies legitimated the barber-surgeon's use of obstetrical forceps and denied midwives the knowledge related to their function, or the legal power to use them, as women were totally barred from using surgical instruments. This legitimated exclusion was coupled with a public campaign, which suggested that if a barber-surgeon with forceps was not present at births then children could die, a point capitalized upon by doctors when they took over the work of barber-surgeons in the eighteenth century. The value of forceps to normal deliveries was never questioned as the implement, and its precise function was shrouded in mystery. As further technical interventions became available for use in difficult childbirths, the mythology that childbirth was a medical problem was developed and maintained.

The reskilling of midwives is a recent phenomena and has occurred as a result of the work of radical feminists who challenged the basis upon which childbirth became medicalized. They set up childbirth processes based on the alternative ideology that childbirth is a natural process (Hirsch 1975; Morgan 1975). The incorporation of this alternate ideology and practices into medicine demonstrates the fragility of some of the claims to superiority upon which medical dominance is founded and the potential of critique to penetrate the myths and to re-create a new construction of reality.

According to Lovell (1980), there is a need to demythologize the practice of medicine. She suggests that medicine has carefully cultivated and capitalized on an image of physicians as priests/gods whose work should not be questioned but who should receive the reverence, respect, and financial rewards that befit the "heros of humanity." She argues that the mythology that has arisen around the practice of medicine means that members of the community are reluctant to challenge medical decisions. However, the very nature of hegemonic relations work to maintain the status quo by supporting the continuance of myths that maintain existing social structures and relationships.

The Effects of Medical Dominance on Nursing

The dominance and power of the medical profession has had important implications for nursing. A brief examination of the recent history of nursing shows its movement from an independent activity carried out by a variety of individuals with no formalized, centralized training or collective identity, to the establishment of a formalized, regulated occupation under the control of medicine.

Florence Nightingale has been identified as the key person in the development of nursing as a subordinate part of the technical division of labor surrounding medicine (Friedson 1970; Pittman 1985). Prior to her reorganization of nursing along hierarchical and military lines, nursing had experienced a history of independence. Nightingale organized her nurses within the framework of military medical camps during the Crimean War and made it a condition that no nurse was allowed to undertake any service without authorization from a doctor. This included such routine tasks as feeding, cleaning, or even soothing a patient, because Nightingale was determined to achieve acceptance for her nurses from the medical profession (Friedson 1970; Dolan 1978). The consequence of this limitation on nursing autonomy was that nursing became a formal part of the doctor's work—that is to say, a "technical trade" (Friedson 1970:61). Therefore, although in the short term nursing was able to organize itself and establish itself as a "full-fledged occupation of some dignity by tying itself to the coat-tails of medicine," in the long term, nursing has struggled with this legacy of medical dominance in order to find a new, independent position in the division of labor (Friedson 1970:63).

Medical dominance is not only apparent in the medical supervision of nursing activities for historic and military reasons but includes the participation by doctors in the role of "experts" in nurse education programs (Reeder 1978). These medical experts were able to make curricula decisions concerning what biophysical and technical knowledge would be useful for nurses. This framing of nursing curricula by doctors maintained the focus of nursing on supporting the needs of the doctors. This enabled doctors to assume control and jurisdiction over nursing activities and the manner in which they are pursued. Doctors defended their role in nursing education on the superiority of their knowledge. This claim was allied with a concern that nurses need to learn to follow medical directions. The necessity for nurses to learn obedience to medical authority was argued on the grounds of patient safety and resulted in a structured subservience that reinforces the dominance of medicine over nursing (Pittman 1985).

To argue that medicine has achieved a position of dominance over nursing is to argue that, through powerful societal
constraints and consensus, nurses have become an oppressed
group and, as such, exhibit characteristics attributable to other
oppressed groups. However, an analysis that views nurses as
an oppressed group does not mean subscribing to a view of a
fixed, unchanging relationship between domination and oppression. Power is not a static phenomena but a process that
depends upon human agency for its relationships and its perpetuation (Foucault 1980a). An analysis of medicine and nursing cannot be reduced to a study in domination or resistance as
there are always moments of cultural and creative expression.
These "moments" are informed by a different logic and constitute true moments of freedom in an otherwise oppressive situation (Giroux 1983). Although nurses generally exhibit the characteristics of an oppressed group, there is also evidence of
moments of resistance and of creative behavior arising out of
different rationales such as gender analysis (Ashley 1980), religious motivation (Dolan 1978), or ethnic or class solidarity
(Thompson 1985).

The medical profession, as the dominant group, has been
able to develop its own norms and values concerning the safe
practice of medicine as the normative ones for the nursing profession and the community. The state supports this hegemony
by the enactment of laws that give the medical profession
power over nursing and, to a lesser extent, other paramedical
professions such as physiotherapy and pharmacy. The nurses
(oppressed) have internalized the image of the doctor (oppressors) and develop a noncritical acceptance of the medical
model as normative (Roberts 1983). This situation is apparent
in some of the moves to develop nursing as a profession that
functions parallel to medicine rather than as a subsidiary
occupation controlled by medicine. Rather than rejecting the
norms and values provided by the oppressors (medicine) in
order to develop the profession of nursing, some nurses have
chosen to use the older established profession of medicine as a
model. Modeling nursing on the the medical model can cripple
the potential for nursing as an emerging discipline with its own
body of knowledge, which is different to, but equally valuable
as medical knowledge.

The acceptance of medical knowledge as normative knowledge means that medical practitioners are socially supported

in their belief in the superiority of medical knowledge over the knowledge of other healthcare providers. They hold positions of authority with health and research funding bodies; therefore, they are able to develop funding guidelines that perpetuate and support research and academic programs that are in the interests of medical dominance. This is evident in situations when research funding bodies are faced with requests for funding from graduate students in nursing, asking research questions about nursing, and judging these proposals by criteria designed only to fit biomedical research. The effect of this is to disadvantage nursing research and to affirm medical practitioners in their beliefs that nurses should be data collectors for medical research rather than active participants in the development of their own body of knowledge. Lack of understanding of qualitative research methods and the questions that they might address leads medical research funding boards to judge qualitative nursing research as "unscientific" and "mickey mouse research." Nurses who want to develop research are often compromised into developing research designs that fit medical expectations rather then focusing on answering nursing questions. This continues the hegemonic control of nursing knowledge by medicine by legitimating medical concerns as the concerns of nursing rather than challenging them.

A further development in nursing that is based on a nursing application of the medical model is the cluster of new occupations that are evolving around nursing—State Enrolled Nurse, physician's assistant, nursing scientists, nurse administrators, nurse educators. Friedson (1970:65) describes the hierarchical nature of this further division of labor as an attempt by nursing to gain status by defining a "subordinate and restricted role...creating a paranursing hierarchy within the paramedical hierarchy." This division of labor in nursing has weakened the overall move towards nursing autonomy because nurses tend to identify with the nursing tasks that they perform rather than with the profession of nursing (Chaska 1978). This identification with the job rather than with a profession has led to a common practice among nurse to be highly mobile—changing jobs frequently looking for better conditions. This behavior has led to the designation of nurses as "touristry" and has focused on the conditions of the workplace rather than on the development of professional skills and knowledge through an ongoing engagement with the practice setting (Friedson 1970).

This adoption of the medical model shows how a potentially counterhegemonic element—the development of nursing autonomy—can be influenced by, and incorporated into, the norms and values of the dominant cultural model of the medical profession. According to Tomich (1978:303), the adoption of the medical model by nursing is "the single most salient and most self-defeating barrier to achievement of full status for nursing as the work of healing." She identifies self-government and self-direction as the two key prerequisites for the achievement of full stature in the division of health labor and believes that a reliance on the medical model implies a lack of self-government and self-direction for nurses. Tomich (1978:303) criticizes the acceptance of the medical model as "a passe overdependency, insecurity in conceptions of the unique services nursing can provide, and a lack of risk-taking in leadership."

Nurses who are successful at assimilating and reproducing the values of the dominant medical profession become "marginal" because of their inability to continue to be representative of the oppressed nursing group and their inability to achieve integration with the medical oppressors (Roberts 1983). They become "adapted" to the values and norms of the dominant medical profession. This attempt to adapt, and the marginal position that it achieves, is evident in the push for an expanded role for nurses. This expanded role means that nurses, particularly in intensive and critical care settings, appropriate areas of medical work that have traditionally been part of the doctor's domain. The development of an expanded nursing role in which well-qualified nurses, particularly those in critical care settings, are taking on roles and functions that rightly belong to the doctor is under contention among some nurses. Lemin (1982:189) says,

> It is clear that nurses are undertaking an expanded scope of practice into areas of questionable legal status. It is clear that an aura of respectability has been given to nurses undertaking these expanded roles by doctors and administrators for the sake of convenience or as the result of bowing to pressure.

While nurses accept these roles for the sake of relationships, status, or concern for the patient, they must recognize that any professionalism they succeed in establishing will be of a second-class nature—if indeed they achieve any professional status in the eyes of healthcare colleagues.

The attempt to assimilate and adapt to the norms of the oppressor leads to a marginal status whereby it is necessary for the oppressed to reject their own characteristics. This rejection of their own nursing characteristics, combined with a failure to be accepted by the dominant medical profession whose characteristics they have adopted, leads to negative feelings about themselves as individuals. Roberts (1983) and Menzies-Lyth (1986) identify these negative personality characteristics in nurses as self-hatred and low self-esteem. They argue that these are commonly found in nurses who undervalue themselves by constantly judging themselves against the adopted normative values of the medical profession and against its accompanying status and prestige. This devaluation of self can lead to feelings of aggression against the oppressor, which must be sublimated to a state of submissiveness in the presence of the aggressor. In nursing this is seen in the doctor/nurse game where nurses disguise their own knowledge and act out a role that supports the myth of the all-powerful, omniscient doctor (Stein 1967).

However, this inability on the part of nurses to oppose the doctors can lead to what Freire (1981) describes as "horizontal violence." This violence is perpetrated by frustrated members of an oppressed group against their peers and becomes the institutionalized oppression of nurses by nurses (Roberts 1983). The relationship between oppression and violence in nursing is described by Lovell (1980:79)

> Once an oppressive relationship is established, violence has already begun. Even when the relationship is sweetened by false generosity it remains oppressive because it does not allow for humanness. People become commodities to be used, abused and manipulated at the whim of the oppressor.

This horizontal violence is practiced by nurses in positions of leadership as these nurses have most successfully adapted to the values and behaviors characteristic of medicine (Roberts 1983). This adaptive behavior is rewarded by the dominant medical profession in ways that lead to leadership within the oppressed area of nursing. The seduction of nurses into an acceptance of the hierarchical relationships instituted by doctors and an imitation of medical roles and values within the field of nursing reduces the need for the doctors, as members of the dominant group, to use coercive power as they can rely on the adapted nursing leaders to maintain their dominant values (Chaska 1978; Monteiro 1978). Nursing leaders do this in order to maintain their own privileges and in a mistaken expectation of sharing power with the oppressors. Cleland (1971) describes these nursing leaders as "Aunt Janes," using the term as a corollary to the "Uncle Tom" label given to adapted black leaders who are supportive of the dominant white culture. These Aunt Janes have been promoted because of their allegiance to the maintenance of the dominant medical and administrative culture. These nurses do not reject the system or the role that male medical administrators and doctors play in the oppression of the largely female nursing profession. They argue that they have reached a position of power and authority in the system and blame their female subordinates for their lack of status.

Within academic settings the rewards that nurses receive for being marginal lead them to support the dominant culture and to argue that it is helpful for clinical nurses to become " bi-cultural" (Roberts 1983). This concept of biculturalism relates to a presumed ability to separate the culture of nursing, as experienced in nursing education, from the medical-based nursing culture of the hospital, and to develop the ability to accept and be accepted equally in each. Roberts argues that this is impossible because nurses, like other oppressed groups, view themselves negatively and reject nursing characteristics of warmth, sensitivity and nurturance when faced with those valued by the dominant medical or educational culture such as intelligence, decisiveness and lack of emotion. In this way nurses are implicated in the oppression of other nurses and maintain a stake in the continuation of the status quo.

4

❧

You Know What Women Are Like!

Nursing probably more than any other occupation except housewifery and prostitution, reflects the stereotyped role of women. The norms and values of nursing are feminine and the relationships between nurses and physicians reflect the extreme subordination of women with all of the male-female games that go along with that subordination.

(Bullough 1975:226)

Gender refers to the social meaning of what it is to be a *man* or a *woman*. Therefore, it includes more than the construction of masculinity and femininity as psychological characteristics—it relates to the more fundamental questions of identity and sexuality. Gender represents a concept of roles of masculinity and femininity that are socially constructed within their relationships to each other (Game and Pringle 1983). Connell (1987) makes this point powerfully when he argues that gender should be regarded as a verb. An understanding of this concept of gendering demonstrate the *a priori* and active element of gender.

The social construction of gender relations in nursing parallels the development of gender relations within society. Feminist analyses of gender relations differ in their theoretical orientations and epistemological claims but share a common commitment to global analyses that value women and their experience, their roles and their contributions to society, along with the identification and confrontation of injustice and

oppression based on gender (Reuther 1975). These feminist
analyses recognize and challenge the ideological component of
gender in the sense that it generalizes from the experience of
one section of society, men, to create an explanation of the
experience of both men and women of the organization of society as a whole, and of the power relations within it. Such an
ideology both denies the experience and objective situation of
women, and justifies the distribution of advantages that arise
from a sexual division, a division which the ideology of patriarchy both ignores and conceals (Roberts 1981:15).

This valuing of women, and the development of systematic
analyses of the consequences for women of a patriarchal society that rewards and values male roles and characteristics, is
vital for nursing. Historically, gender relations in nursing have
been understood as natural and representative of biological
and psychological characteristics between men and women.
Speedy (1987) argues that this legacy continues and is demonstrated in the distrust of feminism expressed by most nurses
and their expression of nursing characteristics in gender-laden
terminology. Implicit or explicit support by nurses for the
maintenance of this deterministic approach facilitates the continued dominance of the class-supported medical model and
militates against the development of nursing autonomy.
According to Rowbotham (1973), determinism is supported by
a male hegemony that limits and influences both the forms
and outcomes of gender struggle.

Game and Pringle (1983:14) challenge the separation of
gender and labor in sociopolitical studies. They believe that
gender is "fundamental to the way work is organized; and work
is central to the construction of gender." Anyon (1984) develops
this focus when she suggests that it is in the intersections of
gender and class that accommodation and resistance to contradictory sex role ideologies can be detected. However, critiques of capitalism generally focus on the sexual division of
labor in terms that differentiate between the home and the
workplace rather than arguing for a sexual division of labor
that also includes the allocation of work, in both the private
and the public spheres, on the basis of sex. Game and Pringle
(1983) have found that the content of men's work and women's
work changes over time and circumstance. They see the stable
factor as the distinction that is made between men's work and
women's work in the context of redefinition of work roles

resulting from technological innovation and bureaucratic structuring. An examination of nursing can demonstrate both the role stereotyping that exists between work and family roles and the way in which these stereotypes are maintained in the face of redefinition of the knowledge, skills, and practices that constitute the doctor/nurse/patient roles.

Family symbolism dominates the nursing literature describing the structuring of medical and nursing roles (Greenleaf 1980; Yeaworth 1978; Bullough 1975). The doctor is represented as the wise powerful father figure who not only has an exclusive access to a elite body of scientific knowledge and the practices that develop from it but whose knowledge, status, and autonomy enable him to benevolently control and direct others. The nurse is represented as the wife who acts in a role that has often been labeled "handmaiden." Her knowledge is the lowly valued practical knowledge, and her role is constructed to carry out the tasks designated by the father/doctor. The child in this symbolic relationship is the patient who is expected to be the passive recipient of the doctor's knowledge and curative practices and of the nurses' caring practices.

The family symbolism is not confined to these individualized relationships but is represented within the institutionalized structures of the hospital. Here the senior medical staff represent the father figure with the director of nursing representing the mother figure who has received a limited realm of authority from the medical staff through which to control the activities of the nursing staff. Symbolically the intern represents the son and heir who is supported and even disciplined by senior nursing staff (aunts) but who is training to inherit the power and prestige of the father/doctor role and to dominate the aunt/charge nurse. Clinical nurses are represented as the daughters, with the patients again assuming the role of the dependant child. Ancillary and support staff become the family servants.

Where has this family symbolism in nursing come from and why does it persist? Although the practice of engaging in informal nursing of relatives in the home by women has been the major form of nursing throughout history, nursing as an occupation was largely carried on by men. Greek priests treated men in their temples or moved with them to nurse them on the battlefield (Dolan 1978). Likewise, the Romans developed tent hospitals and the tent companion (nurse) developed as a specialist role. The medieval period saw the establishment of all-male monastic nursing orders to deal with the wounded Crusaders and the victims of disease. These orders such as the Knights Templars and the Knights of Malta were prestigious orders with systematic knowledge based on herbal remedies. Although these religious orders engaged in both healing and nursing activities, lay women in the community were more often active in occupations related to healing—midwifery, herbalists, witches—than in nursing (Ehrenreich 1973). Female religious orders during this time were generally contemplative enclosed orders, but as the number of female orders multiplied rapidly during the latter middle ages some took on a nursing role. Women taking leadership in convents at this time generally came from wealthy families where informal nursing of vassals and yeomen was carried on by the landed women "noblesse oblige" (Dolan 1978). Industrialization brought changed social roles, overcrowding, plagues, and epidemics meaning that more people required nursing from religious orders of sisters than were available. To fill this need nursing also became the preserve of the lowest level of servants as immortalized by Charles Dickens in the character of the drunken Sairey Gamp in his novel *Martin Chuzzlewit* (1986).

Into this scenario of the now low prestige of secular nurses, and the religious disciplines of poverty, chastity, and obedience that surrounded the religious sisters, came one of the most influential woman in the modern era of nursing—Florence Nightingale. Nightingale changed the status of secular nursing by establishing it as a respectable occupation for women. She was a brilliant woman whose achievements in establishing nursing schools, in research, and in reforming the health conditions of the British army in the Crimea and in India were incredible achievements for a woman in the nineteenth century. However, although Florence Nightingale challenged many of the social stereotypes and created a new role for women as nurses, she also tied their image to the traditional Victorian image of a "good and virtuous woman" (Benjamin and Curtis 1985). As a good Victorian woman Nightingale did not have a highly visible public profile. She withdrew from social life completely after the Crimean War and confined herself to her bedroom, staying there for the next fifty years during which time she received influential, mostly male, admirers and drafted well-researched position papers on a variety of health-related issues. Bullough (1975:227) describes these activities as the work of a "master manipulator who was able to get other people, usually men, to speak for her while she pretended helplessness. Although this strategy was effective for Nightingale, it has had negative consequences for nursing.

Nightingale insisted that nurses should be clean, chaste, quiet, and religious (Nightingale 1859). She agreed with hospital authorities that nurses should work long hours without complaint and be obedient to their nursing superiors and physicians. She was against any self-determination on the part of nurses and fought against the formation of the British Nurses Association (Bullough 1975). Pittman (1985) argues that Florence Nightingale made it plain that nursing did not challenge the authority of the predominantly male medical profession. She described the nursing role as having a function similar to a wife managing a household. She argued that the matron took the role of the wife and supervised all the female hospital staff, but the doctor (father image) made all the decisions on the care of patients. This led to the labeling of nurses as "professional mothers" (Henderson 1978).

However, it is an oversimplification to lay all of the blame for the subordination of nurses on Florence Nightingale, who was a woman of the nineteenth century. Bullough (1975) suggests that the twentieth-century nurses who have uncritically accepted the more repressive assumptions of Nightingale's writings, along with her very real positive contributions, are the real culprits. The lack of analysis of the historical elements in the present nursing theories and practices has allowed the attitudes of the past to define the practice of the present.

Infante (1985) suggests that the history of nursing in developed countries is largely characterized by a reactive rather than an active role in shaping the image of nurses. She argues that since colonial times, female nurses working within the male-dominated area of healthcare have taken cues from nonnurses, notably doctors and administrators, and have yet received from them unquestioned and unequal access to institutionalized status, power, and knowledge. Nurses have tacitly accepted the stereotyping of their nursing role in the same way as women have accepted stereotyping of female roles.

Feminist challenges to the stereotyping of women and women's roles and to the devaluing of characteristics into which females are socialized such as nurturance, collaboration, empathy, and intuition, have taken a variety of forms. Early feminist theories stressed equality of opportunity within the existing social frameworks as the means by which women's oppression would be abolished (Friedan 1963). Nursing analyses based on these insights argued for equality of access to economic rewards, education, research, and administrative opportunities (Chaska 1978). Critique was not aimed at the hegemonic elements of the health system and the prevailing societal attitudes and structures but at the gender discrimination, which prevented nurses from parity and equality within the existing structures of status and power in healthcare. This desire to emulate the oppressor is demonstrated in the development of nursing structures that are based on, and parallel, medical structures, such as nursing diagnoses and nursing prescriptions, an emphasis on the physical sciences in nursing research and education programs. Although this approach may appear to provide access to professional status, and the concomitant advantages of power and status, it forces women to acquiesce to the patriarchal, hierarchical model of medicine and ignores the opportunity to challenge the values and practices of the medical profession despite the increasing questioning of them by the wider community (Wright 1981; Illich 1976). This approach, sometimes labeled liberal feminism, focuses on the rights and opportunities of the nurse with an implicit assumption that better educated nurses who have parity in status and economic rewards with doctors will provide better patient care within the existing structures (Yeaworth 1978). A common critique of liberal feminism is its genesis in white middle-class hetereosexual Western society, which inculcates an apparent disregard for the women of other classes, ethnicity, and sexual orientation. This disregard can enable a selected group of nurses to achieve career goals through the hierarchies of the present system while contributing to the oppression of other staff, ancillary staff, and child care providers whose poorly paid work sustains the professional development of the few. The questions that are neither raised nor addressed within the liberal feminist approach to nursing are the questions of whether nursing that is based on the medical model provides the best patient care, and the more fundamental question of what it is that nursing claims it has to offer to patients and other healthcare providers.

In the United States, where the medical profession competes more openly within its own ranks than in Australia or the United Kingdom, there has been the recent development of the entrepreneurial private nurse who is attempting to "beat the doctors at their own game" by practicing privately and independently (Chaska 1978). These nurses set themselves up in direct competition with the medical profession by advertising their services as a primary focus for community healthcare. These nurse practitioners receive patronage and support from some sections of the community, particularly nurses and feminists, who would rather visit a nurse practitioner for minor illnesses, but, as Friedson (1970) indicates, these nurses still cannot take control of their work in these settings because of their dependence on doctors for pharmaceutical orders. As many of these nurses also rely on good relationships with local doctors and on hospitals, usually governed by male members of the medical profession, the doctor in this process delineates what is nursing practice by virtue of the assignment of tasks to private nurse practitioners. This designation of what tasks doctors allow nurses to carry out means that these nurse practitioners are not developing autonomy from doctors but are being tolerated because they generally attract patients with noncritical illnesses such as viruses. By caring for the nondramatic and noncritical illnesses, these nurses may be doing the doctor and the community a favor. This is indicated by the fact that doctors do refer patients to them but it is the doctor who generally decides what categories of care are needed for the patient, whether a registered nurse, domiciliary care or personal care attendant, and so retains overall control of the patients that he refers. Therefore, something that claims to be offering an autonomous service can in fact be coopted into becoming another aspect of medical service that is under the ultimate control of the doctors. Tomich (1978) is critical of these nurse practitioners who receive reinbursement on a fee-for-service basis as reflecting a relatively uncritical adoption of a medical position that is related to the escalation of healthcare costs. She sees this as a self-defeating action might work to the detriment of nursing. This movement appears to provide a clear example of the way in which a potentially counterhegemonic element is accommodated and incorporated into the dominant culture. This oppositional behavior has made a change in the dominant culture by virtue of its creation of a new role for nurses and an alternative form of healthcare for the community. However, the dominant medical culture has adapted to accommodate the change in such a way that at present the influence of the nurse practitioner movement on the delivery of healthcare services is negligible.

Marxist feminists have challenged the basis of capitalism in which the means of production is controlled by a powerful minority male elite. These critiques generally focus on the sexual division of labor in terms that differentiate between the home and the workplace, between activities of reproduction and activities of production (Hartsock 1983). Nursing analyses influenced by Marxist feminist critique work to uncover the relationship between the traditional stereotyping of the nursing role with that of women generally who are socialized to reproduce the people and the culture of the community (Yeaworth 1978). The activities of production (work) provide access to status in the community and financial rewards through work. Self-worth becomes closely associated with the status that society accords to a particular job and to the salary resulting from that work. Feminist critiques challenge the societal definition of work which is based on occupational and career role and ignores family and domestic roles or community volunteer roles.

Yeaworth (1978) suggests that nursing has provided a part-time occupation for large numbers of women and a career for a few. As a result of this orientation, she believes that nursing has been effective in maintaining the status quo and in remaining a predominantly female occupation tied to the "image of the nurse as the nurturing, feminine, self-sacrificing person who meets the needs of others" (Yeaworth 1978:73). Women may be educated for occupations or even careers in nursing, but they are still effectively socialized to be wives and mothers. Pittman (1985) supports the idea that nursing has been seen as a good preparation for women's traditional roles as wife and mother, and it is seen primarily as "women's work." She writes:

Girls are still socialized to accept subservient roles and many women are actively discouraged from seeking responsible and challenging jobs in occupations dominated by men. (Pittman 1985:12)

Yeaworth sees this socialization process as equipping women, and society, to an expectation that the wife-mother role will be the norm for adult women despite the fact that improved household technology, reduced family size, and changes in social and sexual ideologies may mean that the wife-mother role fills only a small portion, or none, of a women's life. This socialization assumes a caring, nurturing role for all females despite their interests, abilities, or marital situation. Greenleaf (1980) argues that this situation stems from an ideology that defines man's domain as the public sphere and women's as the private sphere, the home. This ideology assumes that all women are supported within families and enter the labor market only to earn pocket money rather than "real" wages. This ideology shapes the realities and demands of the world of wage work against the assumed standard of the male worker. Women, viewed primarily as nonmarket labor, find themselves in marginal positions in the workplace. In nursing this marginality is evident in the high percentage of nurses taking casual work with private agencies to fit in with home and family roles (Game and Pringle 1983). Nurses not only work "double time"—within the home and within the healthcare setting—but find that in both spheres their roles are socially constructed and constrained to the socially devalued area of reproduction. Radical feminist critiques argue that the means of production and reproduction must be shared throughout the whole community and not reside within a particular class or gender group (Hartsock 1983). This kind of radical social restructuring is not a popular option with nurses in Australia (Speedy 1987). It appears that the double oppression that nurses experience, as women and as nurses, maintains an ideological blindness that disguises the gender-based subtext under the nurse/mother role. However, nursing unions do use Marxist feminist critique as the basis for their argument that reproductive activities are as socially useful as productive activities and so should receive equal remuneration and status.

Neo-Marxist feminists and socialist feminists support the need for social restructuring but suggest that Marxist class analysis needs to be supported by analyses of other cultural institutions that oppress women—the family, motherhood, housework, and schools. These analyses recognize the oppression of reproductive activities by productive activities but also argue that reproductive activities are constructed in ways that oppress the participant. The development of analyses on the oppressive nature of housework have informed nursing critiques on the nature of the nursing role which contains a significant number of tasks that can be categorized as housework

(Game and Pringle 1983). These critiques led to the designation of specific tasks as nonnursing duties, which were then delegated to nonnursing personnel such as nursing assistants and cleaners.

Although most gender analysis of nursing focuses on the male/female, dominator/dominated relationship (Chaska 1978; Pittman 1985; Cleland 1971), a number of analyses (Bullough 1975; Greenleaf 1980; Yeaworth 1978) are recognizing that power relations in hospitals are complex and that many female nurses enjoy the power of their positions to the detriment of other women doctors, nurses, nursing aides, cleaners, and, as Evers (1981) found in a geriatric hospital, female patients. This critical work recognizes the "oppressor in the oppressed" (Freire 1972). Nurses as members of an underprivileged group strive to join the more acceptable and privileged medical group and so "develop a negative chauvinism toward their own group and thus de-emphasize the underprivileged group's positive qualities" (Greenleaf 1980:30).

Evers (1981:108) describes the complexity of the problem of being female in a female-dominated but male-subjugated profession, in her research into the treatment of geriatric patients. She found that

> neither in its policy nor in its professional practice does the health-care system take any explicit account of the distinctive characteristics of women geriatric patients. This has adverse consequences for both women patients and nurses. The women patients tend to be subjected to particular forms of oppression: the nurses—also women on the whole—tend to label women patients as more 'difficult' than men. This labeling goes hand in hand with various conflicts for the nurses, who are socialized into a female-dominated 'caring' profession, yet at the same time are subject to administrative pressures towards efficient control of work, by routinising the running of the ward. In the context of these conflicts, the 'difficult ' patient represents both a care problem and a control problem for the nurse.

However, Greenleaf (1980:26) cautions that those involved in seeking an explanation for occupational segregation within nurses often implying deficits in women, in general, that need to be remedied. This kind of approach blames the victim (Ryan

1971) by suggesting a remedial aid, such as workshops on communication, management skills, and assertiveness training, rather than examining the political and social nature of the work. Greenleaf (1980) quotes the work of Kanter on women's disadvantage with respect to organizational power. She has found that power or the lack of it has a great deal of influence on leadership style and that women in institutions are generally channeled into leadership positions that are not organizationally powerful. The derogatory stereotypes of women leaders or bosses stem primarily from the lack of organizational power of their positions. Greenleaf argues that when nurses say, "Nurses are their own worst enemies," they fail to acknowledge the social structure of the situation and how this impinges on the individual. She found that "much of the behavior attributed to women in the workplace emerges as behavior characteristic of stuckness, for men who are stuck exhibit the same tendencies" (1980:26).

An analysis of the oppression of nurses takes up the points made by Ryan (1971) in relation to the tendency to devalue the victims of oppression. Greenleaf (1980:33) argues that

> to view the segregation of any non-dominant group as having only negative effects on its members is to ignore tremendous contributions that have come to us from oppressed people throughout history...This is not to suggest that oppression and its effects should be idealized, but rather to point out that the oppression of one human group by another does indeed exist and understanding the processes by which oppressed groups endure and contribute to the overall society is an important step in a fuller appreciation of our humanity.

This kind of argument contains an important insight into the worth of people who are oppressed and their capacity for creativity in their social relationships. However, this process of affirmation can be counterproductive in that it is a short step to a functionalist position which accepts, albeit grudgingly, a society containing oppressors and oppressed. A more helpful analysis for nursing would include a critique of oppression and resistance that recognizes not only a moment of domination but also the possibility for the oppressed to produce, reinvent, and create the ideological and material tools they need to break through the myths and structures that prevent them from transforming an oppressive social reality (Giroux 1983).

Speedy (1987) suggests that this kind of analysis is very difficult for nurses who are socialized into a traditional female gender role that is mimicked within their work role. She believes that nurses accept liberal feminist positions, which enable them to argue for parity with the male-dominated medical profession, but reject Marxist, socialist, and neo-Marxist feminist positions with their focus on the need to overthrow existing social systems, which are based on a male-defined reality. According to Chinn (1985) and Speedy (1987), nurses perceive that the redefined social reality of these feminist groups will be antimale and promoting lesbianism. As Chinn (1985) reminds us, the formation of knowledge, theories, and ideologies that stem from and value the experience of women, is not equivalent to holding a position which devalues men.

In contrast to these feminist analyses, which share a common perspective that defines and values women in relation to men and from this develop alternatives to patriarchal systems, are the radical feminists who develop their analyses from a different premise. They reject the notion that changes to class and economic systems will eliminate the oppression. In an attempt to bypass male ideological values and structures, they seek to develop cultural and theoretical perspectives of a worldview centered on women. Within nursing these alternatives formulate women's health issues and needs. The self-care women's health movement provides a direct challenge to the power of the medical profession and its philosophical underpinnings (Hackett 1977). This movement represents an area of resistance in women's health because it rejects the paradigm on which the medical model is based and develops a competing paradigm to critique and redefine health and illness. This area is relatively new, and although it has received some support and interest from feminist nurses, it suffers from being labeled "deviant" by mainstream members of the nursing profession whose focus is on technology and by members of the community. This labeling has tended to isolate nurses and feminists from each other and from access to publication of deviant views in mainstream media (Spender 1981). However, the mere existence of the deviant label serves to demonstrate that the proponents of this view have been successful in resisting cooption by the medicalized view of healthcare.

This valuing of women's experience will conflict with cultural and nursing values. There is a cultural consensus that altruism and the roles of caregivers are essential for the general well-being of the community and its members (Oakley 1986). These roles serve the community in important ways, but often the altruistic caring individuals are not perceived to be important in themselves. Oakley (1986) contends that women who live altruistic lives or work in occupations where altruism is important generally have low self-esteem. The important caring roles in Western culture are done by women who recognize the sociocultural necessity of these roles but experience the contradictions when these roles are not accorded the political, social, economic, and cultural valuing that is accorded to roles and community contributions culturally assigned to men. Nurses, like mothers, experience this as a dichotomy. Their experience of providing nursing care affirms its value but the experience of participating in a male-dominated healthcare system that values "cure" over "care" devalues nursing and disadvantages nurses. The symbolic role of the nurse receives general community adulation but the reality of being a nurse demonstrates the illusionary nature of the cultural commitment to caring roles. According to Dunlop (1986), the concept of caring carries an etymological legacy of negative associations that are difficult to isolate and challenge because they are so culturally embedded. Nurses in low-status caring roles are faced with the dilemma of doing good while feeling bad. Clinical roles that facilitate patient communication, advocacy, and autonomy are devalued daily by the societal valuing of complex technological, medical interventions.

Feminist nurses such as Roberts (1981), Lovell (1980), and Greenleaf (1980) have written about the positive aspects of the feminine role.Some attributes that nurses as women possess may have been perceived in the past as inappropriate and incongruent with creativity but are becoming more accepted in today's society. For example, nurses as women have been described as intuitive, usually framing the world in a context that compares it with more prestigious male-defined values such as rationality. Benoliel (1975) suggests that increasingly, as Eastern and Western modes of knowledge development and merge, intuition is being seen in a more positive light as a component in different patterns of understanding reality and as a method for scientific inquiry. She argues that powerless women such as nurses perceive reality differently to those who occupy positions of social power and dominance, yet their perceptions have much to contribute to knowledge about nurturance and the care-taking process. Styles (1982) argues that nurses need to develop and affirm these so-called feminine attributes of caring, collegiality, and cooperation. She exhorts nurses to believe in themselves and in their colleagues as a basis for the development of professional collegial relationships.

The work of feminist nurses such as Keen (1988) and Wheeler and Chinn (1989) have provided nursing with challenges to critique and reconstitute the basis of these professional collegial relationships through processes that critique patriarchy and affirm the specific values of caring and friendship between nurses. Keen (1988:29–30) challenges the oppressive practices of nurses, which support horizontal violence, and reflects upon the nature of female nursing friendships in the context of being a nurse when she writes:

Every time I am tempted to go and sell real estate instead of being a nurse, it helps me to recall that the neatest, most centred, most loving, caring people that I know in the world are nurses. In my childhood, one woman showed me a different way of being. She was a nurse and I wanted to be like her, so I chose nursing as a career. In my adult life, women—mainly my nursing friends from school and work, have been there to help me through the hard times. They've also come together to create and share some of the best times in my life. Our network of caring remains strong, even though we now live all over the country and can't see each other very often. I don't think my friends are unique, even though stereotypes (those voices from the patriarchy) continue to enforce the notion that women don't generally like each other.

By writing of her experiences of sharing her life with caring nursing friends, Keen seeks to validate her own experience of being a nurse and of being a woman. She asserts that this validation needs to be made consciously and continually in order for nurses to undo and unlearn the oppressive processes that have shaped their lives as women and as nurses.

Connell (1987) describes these strategies as *liberated zones*, a term he uses not only apply to a separatist physical

space but to the *social spaces* created by networks of relationships that resist the dominant sexist ideologies. He argues that
these liberated zones are hard to maintain because the require
greater commitment and energy while receiving less resources
and structural support from conventional institutions. However, these costs are offset by gains in the provision of bases for
wider political scope; through opportunities to engage in experiencing elements of a visionary hope in the activities of the
present; and the support networks to help conserve personal
energy and repair the damage sustained through constant
exposure to oppressive ideological practices.

I would assert that these concepts need careful attention
if nurses are to reflect upon and change the gendered structuring of their nursing role in ways that are empowering for themselves, their colleagues and, in particular, for the healthcare of
the community.

5

🎈

Forget the Study—Real Nursing Is Learned on the Job

...why is it that some skeptics in nursing are still saying, in the latter part of the 20th century, that theory or theorizing in nursing is antithetical to the practice of nursing, that nursing practice is either a practically or theoretically oriented situation and therefore that choosing one standpoint leaves no room and no need for the other?

(Meleis 1985:36)

This question divulges the continuing theory/practice gap in nursing, which is based on the belief that clinical nurses engage in nursing actions and nurse scholars theorize about nursing actions. In her argument for the development of theoretical nursing, Meleis (1985) claims that nursing has moved forward from the historical tendency to divorce theory from practice to a position that accepts the varied meanings of experience as the basis for knowledge development but also accepts that interpretation and analysis of the data experienced is conducted in a form which is *a priori*. This *a priori* construction through which knowledge about nursing is developed is generally designated as a paradigm.

A "paradigm" embodies the particular conceptual framework through which the community of researchers operates and in terms of which a particular interpretation of 'reality' is generated. It also incorporates models of research, standards, rules of inquiry and a set of techniques and methods, all of which ensure that any theoretical knowledge that is produced will be consistent with the view of reality that the paradigm supports. (Carr and Kemmis 1983:72)

Meleis's (1985) contention concerning the new directions in the development of nursing theory rests on her identification of varying paradigms being used by nursing scholars to develop nursing knowledge. These paradigms are evident within the academic community of nurses but are often used to support or enhance knowledge developed through the dominant positivist paradigm.

Polkinghorne (1983:203) describes knowledge acquired through this positivist paradigm as *formal*—it describes facts or events in terms of formal properties; *theoretical*—it derives from knowledge obtained by an observer who is disengaged from the world being observed; *functional*—it uses mathematics to relate abstract elements in terms of their functional relationships; and *quantitative*—in that the research material is organized and categorized in numerical relationships.

The Development of Nursing Scholars

A journey of exploration into the territory of nursing practice will be a journey that is shaped by the theoretical interests brought by the researcher to the clinical context and the theoretical interests that inform the nursing action the researcher finds there. It is, therefore, useful to chart the development of nursing knowledge, pursuing the relationships between its interests and the methods and interests of the positivist paradigm.

It would be simplistic to suggest that nursing scholarship has progressed tidily through stages that build on each other. In nursing, as in other academic areas, there have always been those who have dissented from the normative paradigm. For the ease of this discussion I have represented the growth of positivism as the dominant paradigm for nursing in a series of stages. These stages overlap and continue concurrently. All these stages have affected some nurse scholars so that nursing research mirrors the messy nature of other academic research in its adherence to particular expressions of either a positivist or alternative perspective.

Historically nursing has been considered an occupation based on caring and simple curative practices. Yet the scientific explosion of the nineteenth century developed knowledge in anatomy, physiology, and the biological sciences, which has dramatically affected the healthcare practices of all healthcare providers. The modern nurse is no longer expected only to provide basic bedside care as nursing practice has been revolutionized by the use of the products of the scientific explosion—high technology and drugs (Willis 1983). Nurses have been required to acquire a basic mastery of the appropriate areas of the physical sciences to provide safe healthcare (Henderson 1980). This emphasis on the need for greater scientific and technological understanding for nurses has led increasing numbers of nurses to participate in higher education programs, which will equip them with the requisite scientific and technical knowledge. These higher degree courses have introduced them to the paradigm and methodology of the natural sciences. Therefore, nursing has not only adopted the products and knowledge of the natural sciences in the practice of nursing, but of the *positivist* or *empirical* paradigm of research, theory building, and the applied view of knowledge used by the scientific community (Silva 1984).

According to Thompson (1985), positivism has had a profound effect on the development of nursing scholarship. She suggests that Popper's argument that the scientific method is concerned not with confirmation but with a rigorous attempt to falsify hypotheses led the way for the acceptance of the "proper" scientific method to be utilized to develop knowledge about nursing. Both Silva (1984) and Thompson (1985) argue that this stage of development is still present in nursing in the shape of theoretical discourse over the proper techniques for analyzing concepts. These nursing scholars focus their attention on research activities that facilitate the semantic analysis of words and concepts and on the techniques for operationalizing them.

This kind of semantic analysis is apparent in the work of many nursing scholars who are convinced that there must be permanent, ahistorical standards for grounding knowledge in reality. Positivists argue that if concepts are defined clearly and distinctly enough, and if they are linked to corresponding pieces of reality, they can serve as fundamental epistemological units, as a stable, unchanging foundation for future knowledge

claims. According to Thompson, these attempts by nurse scholars to isolate logical proper names and to use rigorous methods
for definitions are in reality this kind of search for foundations.

In the mid 1960s nurses who were interested in teaching
or research received their graduate education in programs outside the discipline of nursing. To do so nurses moved from
their female-dominated undergraduate programs to the male-
dominated graduate programs of the natural sciences and education. Many of these nurses accepted the dominant positivist
paradigm and the scientific method without question (Munhall
1982). They became increasingly involved with hypotheses
testing and, as independent nursing research departments
developed, many areas of nursing scholarship continued to
cling to this focus despite changes in positivist methodology
(Thompson 1985).

As nurse scholars began to engage in theory development,
many began to examine the relationship between theory and
practice in an attempt to develop theory that was more relevant
to practice. The work on the development of nursing theory
(practice theory) pioneered by Dickoff and James, and imitated
by many nurse researchers, is based on the need to explain
nursing practices and to develop nursing prescriptions (Dickoff
1968). However, Thompson (1985) contends that practice theory is no more than the formalization of a popular view of
hypotheses testing in nursing. O'Toole (1981:12) supports the
work by Dickoff and James on practice theory arguing that
"prescriptive theory has particular utility in nursing." She continues to be committed in her support for positivist research for
nursing despite evidence from clinical nurses involved in her
own research who suggest that it is inappropriate. In her words:

> Perhaps another reason for the deficit in practice research
> is that clinicians find the intuitive approach to patient
> care to be creative and thus gratifying, and the structured
> and systematic approach of research to be stifling."
> (O'Toole 1981:17)

As a way of attempting to deal with this contradiction
O'Toole argues that the paucity of studies about practice might
be related to the lack of technological sophistication in practice
interventions. This is a common complaint by nurse scholars
who are frustrated in their efforts to gain support for experi-

mental research into practice from practitioners who do not see any value in the research. Nurse scholars, such as Winstead-Fry in 1980, were attempting to utilize the reductionist scientific method to develop nursing research on holistic health while acknowledging the difficulties equating objectivity with holism. A common response to the inadequacies experienced by zealous researchers dominated by the desire to produce rigorous scientific research on nursing practice was to "blame the victim" (Ryan 1971). In this way nurses are blamed for their inability to use the scientific method properly rather than subjecting the model to scrutiny and questioning its suitability as a means for nurses to engage in research on nursing practice

With the progression in nursing scholarship, discourse in nursing demonstrates an empirical shift from isolated hypotheses testing based on isolated propositions, words, or sentences to a new focus on a conceptual scheme or framework (Rogers 1980 & 1981; Roy 1980, 1981). The work of Roy, Rogers, and other nurses has led to the development of a number of conceptual schemes that are being used as the basis for discourse and testing (Meleis 1985; Barclay 1986). These conceptual frameworks generally consist of diagrams, words, and sentences arranged together to depict a conceptual scheme. These conceptual frameworks are often confused with theory development, which is the process of thinking about and reflecting on nursing practice. Bernstein (1983:75) responds to these confusions when he confesses to

> ...deep difficulties in trying to clarify just what is a conceptual scheme, how we demarcate one conceptual scheme from another and how radical are the differences among various conceptual schemes. But an even more fundamental difficulty concerns what these so-called conceptual schemes are supposed to be about.

Meleis (1985) suggests that the use of "conceptual frameworks" has been a substitute for theory development in nursing. She describes the dilemmas faced by students in the United States, who were taught to think of nursing practice as a series of interrelated concepts, as

> a decade that overwhelmed students with esoteric content rarely used in practice after graduation...the schism that

existed between the language of clinicians and educators
had convinced students of the uselessness of the esoteric
content even before their own graduation and entry into
the work force. (Meleis 1985:45)

She contends that the focus on conceptual frameworks for
nursing scholars caused them to be

...lulled into thinking that using conceptual frameworks
was the way to develop theories and theoretical thinking.
Therefore, focus on conceptualizing curricula caused us
to lose sight of the reason for it in the first place: nursing
practice. (Meleis 1985:46)

Silva *(1984)* suggests that it is ironic that at the time these
conceptual frameworks were beginning to make a profound
impression on nursing, the positivist view expressed in them
was undergoing a strong repudiation from many philosophers
of science. She argues that the relative isolation of many nurse
researchers in schools of nursing, removed from the mainstream of academic thought, gave them a heavy reliance on the
scientific method in which they had received their graduate
training. Therefore, the development of conceptual models to
describe and predict nursing care, while being useful in providing a variety of systematic ways of viewing nursing, is unable to
answer all the needs of the clinical nurse in practice who with
Meleis (1985) finds it difficult to look at "a nursing client as an
energy field, a system of behavior, or a self-care agent."

The next stage—the postempiricist stage—is the move from
theory and concept testing to an understanding of the conflict
between different theories, developed out of different paradigms,
and of the role of the historical development in the formulation
of a research program (Thompson 1985). This interest in his-
toricity represented a move in thinking that confronted the normative ways of developing knowledge about nursing.

The challenges of some nurse scholars to the normative
paradigm worked to define the limits of that paradigm and
opened the way for paradigmatic shifts to occur. An interesting
report on positivist research in nursing that highlights this
growing self-consciousness described by Thompson, is the
work of Patricia Munhall (1982). She revisits a study that she
had conducted earlier, using the empirical method, on the

moral development of nurses. She acknowledges that at the inception of the original study she did not question either the theory presented by Kohlberg or the validity of the scientific method to prove her hypothesis. She states that she was able to produce evidence to support her case that ethics should be taught to student nurses. She had unquestioningly accepted both the limits of the theory and the paradigm in which the theory was constructed. However, the influence of feminist research and grounded theory on Munhall's work meant that she began to engage in a "critical self-appraisal" of her conclusions, of the theory, and of the paradigm in which the research process had been located. This fresh approach led her to unravel a number of methodological fallacies in her research and to argue strongly against the use of empirical methods in nursing research on clinical practice.

As Munhall stretched the limits of the paradigm and then moved beyond them to advocate an alternative paradigm, she offered a strong challenge to those nurse scholars who were working with the dominant paradigm. This action elicited two oppositional responses. Munhall received affirmation from other nurse scholars who were also engaging in challenging the limits and scope of the dominant paradigm and moving towards their own paradigmatic shifts. She also received a defensive response from nurse scholars such as Gortner (1983), who argued that empirical, scientific methods have resulted in good research by nurses. By good Gortner means that nurses have developed mastery of the scientific method and are able to produce highly proficient experiments. Fawcett (1984:9) supported this claim and, building on the work of Gortner, she argued that problems have arisen when

nurses have expected nursing research to have immediate applicability for practice...In other disciplines, it is a well-known fact that the actual use of research findings often is decades after generation of basic research findings.

Neither Fawcett or Gortner explain how nurses can go about finding answers to problems that arise for them in practice. They expect nurses to feed their problems to nursing researchers for research and later (in fact, much later) publication as a basis for application by clinical nurses. This contention is consistent with their adherence to the dominant paradigm, which like any other paradigm can be defended against challenges by recourse to its own set of criteria for viewing the world.

The backlash, typified by Gortner and Fawcett, against challenges to the positivist paradigm of research in nursing indicates that this paradigm is still the normative one for nursing research. Nevertheless there are an increasing number of nurses who are recognizing the limitations of the positivist method for research into nursing practice (Benner 1984; Chaska 1978; Daubenmire 1973; Henderson 1977, 1980; Wilson 1977; Simms 1981; Silva 1984; Reeder 1978; Pearsall 1965; Carper 1978; Yeaworth 1978).

Clinical Nurses and the Development of Nursing Knowledge

The moves to explore alternative paradigms have developed in response to an increasing concern over the irrelevance and inaccessibility of knowledge, derived from the positivist paradigm, for clinical nurses. This oversubscription to externally derived understandings of practice has meant that the richness and intrinsic realities embedded in clinical practice are ignored and devalued. According to Moss (1987), the culturally embedded effect of this devaluation of clinical practice is the most important issue before Australian nurses at the present time. She argues that it is essential for nursing to develop a paradigmatic shift towards nursing practice.

Meleis (1985:51) examines the work of nurse scholars and argues that the old paradigms of knowledge are being challenged by a shift to include

> humanitarianism, holism, the incorporation of sociocultural content, perceptions of subjects of research, subjects and researchers collaborating in the research process, and a qualitative approach....

She contends that these paradigmatic shifts are developing in response to a changed worldview that

> is congruent with women's views of science and nurses' view of health. It is a view that has shifted the focus from the causation to a more interpretive view. It is heightened by phenomenology and qualitative research.

According to Meleis these paradigmatic shifts are moving nurses into a search for a common language to describe patient care and patient outcomes. She sees this quest for better communication about clinical practice as a quest for theory development. In this way Meleis differentiates between the distinctive features of theory and practice while arguing for their interrelationship.

Feminist nurses suggest that, despite being created by female nurses, most of these conceptual frameworks use "man" as a generic concept although this practice is untenable from sociological, psychological, and linguistic frames of references. Therefore, these conceptual frameworks have not only been constructed by nurses, whose higher degree work has been conducted within male-dominated physical and natural sciences utilizing the positivist paradigm, but have generalized from the experiences of illness in males to encompass the experiences of illness in females.

Feminists have opened the door to questions which are of significance to women's health needs; this has often corresponded with an interest in the phenomena of nursing that can be known through experience. Nursing scholars have appropriated the philosophical insights of phenomenology, existentialism, structuralism, and dialectics to facilitate an examination of phenomena, such as "empathy," "caring," "languaging," and "transforming," encountered in the lived experience of clinical practice. An interest in understanding these phenomena in relation to nursing has necessitated forays into the realms of philosophical thought and the attendant qualitative methodologies that support examinations of the subjective experiences of being a nurse. Theorists like Moccia (1981), Parse (1981), Leininger (1981), and Watson (1987) have generated their conceptual frameworks from perspectives informed by existentialist phenomenology. These nurses argue that nursing is a human science and as such needs to reject the premises and methods of the natural sciences.

Leininger (1984) claims that the central theme upon which nursing knowledge and nursing practice is predicated is caring. This concern with caring as a central tenet of nursing practice is pursued by Watson (1987) who suggests that clinical nursing can be illuminated through metaphoric vignettes of nursing care. Parse (1981) uses the existentialist phenomenology of Satre, Merleau-Ponty, and Heidegger to evolve a conceptual framework of "Man-Living-Health" (unfortunately she has based this concept on a generic term that is now unacceptable within academic scholarship); however her work demonstrates a commitment to the human interrelationships, which can be addressed in the debate on the direction of nursing knowledge.

Moccia (1988) uses her philosophical stand to argue that questions of ontology, epistemology, values, and intentions need to be attended to by nursing scholars in order to provide a basis for understanding clinical nursing. Moccia argues for the use of dialectics to inform nursing knowledge. The work of Parker (1988) owes a debt to phenomenology and hermeneutics because she argues for nursing to engage with the concepts of *time, place,* and *person* in the project of understanding nursing practice.

These nursing scholars are writing about ways of understanding nursing practice from their academic positions. Benner (1984) reminds us that little is known about the knowledge that clinical nurses have and use because they do not have a tradition that supports the recording of data about practice. This lack of systematic descriptive data about clinical practice impoverishes nursing by disregarding knowledge that develops through time and the experience of nursing. She suggests that nursing scholars have studied nursing practice from the perspectives of role relationships, socialization, and acculturation but have disregarded the domain of knowledge accrued through the practice of nursing. As a consequence nurse scholars treat all nurses as if they are working with the knowledge they gained through their formal education programs and disregard the idiosyncratic, context-specific knowledge gained through prolonged clinical experience. Benner uses Polanyi's (1962) concept to argue that the nurse scholars can "know that" about clinical practice but disregard "know-how" or practical knowledge. Benner's work is based on the work in hermeneutics of Heidegger (1962) and Dreyfus (1980), and she is concerned with the examination of reported situations in clinical practice when experience, defined as "preconceived notions and expectations are challenged, refined, or disconfirmed by the actual situation," develops into clinical expertise (Benner 1984:3). She contends that the knowledge embedded in clinical expertise makes it possible for nurses to interpret clinical situations and engage in complex decision making.

Benner's commitment to hermeneutics and the interpretive paradigm has enabled her to examine the meanings in clinical nursing and to begin to interpret them. Her work has been very influential in nursing in the United States and in Australia and has been copied rather than critiqued (see Dunlop 1986). Using participant observation and interviews Benner limits herself to working with exemplars of clinical expertise. She has used a framework developed by Dreyfus (1980) to categorize the exemplars of clinical situations into competencies ranging from novice to expert. She works with isolated instances of practice and argues that these exemplars do not represent an "expert nurse" but instances of expert practice within the specific context.

As we have seen with other nursing theorists, a key focus of Benner's work is a commitment to the primacy of the phenomenon of caring in the development of nursing knowledge. She suggests that caring in nursing can be understood as practical knowledge, which is obtained by use of the methods of the interpretive paradigm. This moves the focus away from a medical model in which the focus is on curing the patient. Benner contends that this focus on curing relates to technical knowledge of the kind uncovered by positivist methodology. Benner (1988) does not deny the function of "cure" in the nursing role but argues that the main function of nursing is providing "care." She is careful not to suggest that other members of the healthcare team do not provide care also but contends that nursing is based on the primacy of caring. This focus has received some critique from nurses in areas such as intensive care who argue that patients come into hospital expecting interventions that will cure their condition and not primarily to receive care. Others who have been influenced by Benner have tried to frame caring within a positivist framework and ask questions such as, "Is a science of caring possible?" (Dunlop 1986:661)

The care/cure debate has generally been conducted within nursing academia as a response to nursing's historical reliance on the medical model focused on cure. However, very little has been documented of the work of clinical nurses and the ways in which they make sense of technical and practical knowledge. Benner's method of isolating specific instances of practice from the socially and historically constructed contextual daily routines of a nursing shift provides some documentation of clinical knowledge, but it ignores issues that constrain and shape clinical practice. She suggests that examinations of nursing should be "conducted by self-interpreting subjects (researchers) who are studying self-interpreting subjects (participants) who both may change as a result of an investigation" (Benner 1984:171, original emphasis). Therefore, Benner's key concern is with understanding and valuing nursing practice, but in the process it can be argued that she disregards the politics of power at work in nursing.

Nurse Scholars and the Examination of Power and Knowledge in Clinical Nursing

According to Thompson (1985), interpretive and holistic methods enable nurses to address the historical and traditional prejudices that direct nursing but fail to confront the material, social, and political conditions as sources of domination and authority in nursing. She suggests that it would be valuable for nurses to move beyond positivist and interpretive paradigms and explore knowledge that arises from a critique of domination. She advocates that nurses should begin to look toward the work of Habermas (1971, 1973a) for an understanding of the ways in which interpretations of meaning and context can be distorted by processes of power.

In her study, on the implications of technology on nursing in Australia, Brewer (1986:91) found that most nurse educators and nursing administrators did not believe that clinical nurses were using technical or practical theory in nursing practice. They believed that there were historical, hierarchical, institutional, and gender constraints that shaped nursing practice. Perry (1987:6) argues that it is

> becoming increasingly difficult for nurses to both hold expert clinical knowledge, and to act on that knowledge in a clinical setting within an institution.

She suggests that nurses are socialized into an acceptance of taken-for-granted practices, institutional rules, and routines, which enable them to participate willingly in their own domination (Perry 1986). Perry contends that this socialization is a political process that needs to be critiqued using critical theory in order to demonstrate the power relations at work in the development of nursing knowledge.

In summary, nursing literature describes a long history of technical nursing knowledge developed through variations on the dominant positivist paradigm. During the last decade paradigmatic shifts have occurred with some nurses beginning to use a variety of alternative methods to develop practical knowledge through theory and methods that can loosely be described as belonging to a interpretive paradigm, which includes liberal feminist critiques. There is considerable confusion of methods and theory in nursing paradigms with evidence of research being based on interpretive paradigms, including empirical work done to validate the research (e.g., Pearson 1985). This points to lack of clarity in understanding the theoretical bases of the varying paradigms and the hegemonic power of the dominant positivist paradigm in nursing. This is evident in the manner in which the methodology of action research, which in Australia is usually associated with a critical paradigm analyzing power relations, has been coopted as a methodology for introducing hierarchical institutional changes in nursing (Hunt 1987; Pearson 1985; Bailey and Claus 1975) and developed as an "applied" strategy for change.

However, the situation in nursing scholarship is changing rapidly and, although current nursing journals demonstrate the primacy of the positivist paradigm for nursing throughout the English-speaking world, many nurses emerging from graduate programs are using alternative paradigms to inform their, yet unpublished, work. Some nurse scholars are arguing for the examination of critical theory as a paradigm for the development of nursing knowledge. According to Allen (1985), nursing research needs to recognize the relationships between forms of research and the forms of knowledge that they develop. He argues that the dominant empirical-analytical form of research is determined by a fundamental interest in control and needs to be challenged when the nursing research interest is in issues of empowerment. Although as yet there is very little substantive work published in this area, Perry and Moss (1988) have developed the diploma of nursing curriculum for Deakin University's School of Nursing using the theoretical insights of Habermas's concept of knowledge—constitutive interests as an organizing framework. This curriculum is already making an impact among nurses interested in understanding and changing the culture of nursing. Through emerging courses, which provide a diversity of academic and research views, an increasing number

of undergraduate and graduate nursing students in Australia
are being prepared to engage with the domain of critical social
theory and the reflective processes that support this philosophical and theoretical stance.

Nurses are becoming aware that whereas technical and
practical knowledge can provide knowledge for use by nurses
and can provide sociocultural knowledge about practice, these
kinds of knowledge can also support the status quo by ignoring the class, gender, and power relations at work in healthcare. Therefore, some nursing scholars are beginning to look
towards neo-Marxist and radical feminist theory and critical
theory as a basis for the development of empowering nursing
knowledge (Chinn 1985; Speedy 1987; Thompson 1985; Perry
1985, 1986, 1987).

The work of feminist nurses such as Hedin and Duffy
(1988) are leading the way in developing research structures
that are reflective of their feminist stance. These research processes share a common agenda with critical approaches in
their commitment to the values of

> an emancipatory interest: the aim is enlightenment and
> more specifically, the empowerment of women and the
> transformation of patriarchal structures and relations that
> perpetuate the oppression of women. (Hedin and Duffy
> 1988:365)

This feminist interest in enlightenment, empowerment,
and emancipation are evident in the work of Wheeler and
Chinn (1989:1) who use the acronym PEACE in order to explicate the values of Praxis, Empowerment, Awareness, Consensus, and Evolvement. Other nurses are looking to the work of
ecofeminists in order to develop a perspective on nursing that
takes account of ecological, cosmological, and spiritual values
in relation to healing and the nursing role. Another interesting
dimension, which is being given attention in the move to develop nursing knowledge, is the move towards artistic, aesthetic,
and intuitive ways of making sense of the healthcare world and
of being a nurse situated within it.

These forms of knowledge creation, which challenge the
domination of the normative paradigms for understanding
nursing, are pregnant with exciting possibilities of dreams,
which can be translated into action that is transformative and
healing for our whole society.

6

🍂

Reading the Map Symbols:
Key Concepts

Any study purporting to examine the lived experiences of people needs to take account of the need to define and elaborate the theoretical content of key words and concepts used as the basis for the analysis. My commitment to the concept of the constitutive nature of language means that a shared understanding of the meanings expressed is essential to the development of my argument.

Culture

A general definition of culture suggests that it represents human action and its products, which are socially constructed and transmitted (Mitchell 1968). Williams (1977:19) highlights the historical contribution of Marx to a changed understanding of culture, which rejects as incomplete the notion of "people making their own history" through a focus on the history of religion and states, and moves to a concept of culture that includes the material history of labor, of "people making themselves" through producing their own means of life.

A concept of culture that includes human action, experience, and material production is inevitably related to dynamics of power. Therefore, culture is a form of production that relates intimately to the structuring and mediating of social processes, and the transforming action of language and resources in resisting and reconstituting them. Culture is never static or homogeneous. It is enacted in asymmetrical relationships, which reflect the struggles and contradictions between individuals and groups in the elaboration of and production of social formations and goals. Within a particular culture different groups represent different interests with differential access to status and power. This differential access is reflected in hierarchical relationships between groups and classes in which power is used by a dominant group to consolidate their interests and to convince the subordinate group to consent to the continuation of the existing order. Culture not only includes multiple groups but is also a term which describes particular groups in relation to others. This is the basis on which it is possible to describe nursing culture as a subordinate cultural group in relation to the dominant medical culture. Nursing culture includes practices, beliefs, knowledge, and resources that may accommodate those of the dominant medical culture, resist them, or remain indifferent to them (Giroux 1983).

Ideology

According to Williams (1977), Marxist writings contain three common versions of the concept of ideology. Ideology represents the system of beliefs characteristic of a class or group, the false consciousness or illusionary beliefs that can be tested against rational or scientific knowledge, or the general process by which meanings and ideas are produced. These common versions manifest ideology as both the ideas and the process by which these ideas are created and reproduced.

In this study ideology is taken to represent the concepts, beliefs, and values that characterize a social group and develop and sustain shared meanings through the practices of communication, decision making, production, and reproduction. Ideology critique is the process by which these patterns of shared social meanings are subject to scrutiny with an explicit aim of demonstrating the internal contradictions and false understandings inherent in them.

Hegemony

The traditional meaning of hegemony relates to the concept of political domination or rule in relation to political states. Gramsci cogently (1971) separated "rule," with its overtones of domination by direct action and coercion, from a concept of hegemony, which describes the complex ideological control exercised by the dominant beliefs, attitudes, and codified patterns of social action within interlocking political, cultural, and social formations. In this sense Gramsci argues that hegemony denotes the boundaries of common sense and common concerns for most people and as such can explain the failure of structured oppositional movements to change the balance of power within the hegemonic relationship of dominant and subordinate cultures. Analytically, hegemony denotes an instrument of domination and legitimation in culture that represents the structured inequalities in means and capacities, which are taken-for-granted and constitute social reality for most people. As such, hegemony can be described as a totalizing concept that saturates social understandings to the extent that political, cultural, and social constructions of reality become invisible to most people. This invisibility enables hegemonic relationships to be continually recreated and reconstituted through power and knowledge relationships, which legitimate the dominant group. However, a hegemony of power and knowledge that legitimates the domination of a cultural group is never completely under the control of that group (Giroux 1981). The diversity of ideologies and processes engaged in by subordinate groups provides critical moments, which hold the potential for challenge and change to the existing hegemonic culture. These critical moments occur at points where contradictions, confusion, and discontinuities are evident within the ideological control of the dominant group as ideology critique and structural inconsistencies challenge the hegemony of dominant discourses.

Accommodation

These critical disjunctions can result in accommodation, which represents the process of adjustment engaged in by both the dominant and subordinate groups. In an endeavor to bypass or subjugate overt expressions of hostility between the groups, this process essentially reconstructs the status quo with social, political, or economic concessions made to the subordinate groups. In this way both groups can accept and accommodate concessions and changes without disturbing the basic power or knowledge relationships. This process of accommodation is visible in the contestation that surrounds nursing and medical roles in relation to new technology. As the role of intensive care nurse is redefined through a process of knowledge acquisition and contestation to include technical skills and tasks previously identified as the exclusive domain of doctors, the power and knowledge gap is reconstituted through the rapid acceleration of medical technology. This escalation of medical knowledge and skills in the area of intensive care means that the doctors can accommodate the challenges of nursing by relinquishing control over repetitious or more mundane tasks, such as regular tests to determine the oxygen content in the blood, without reducing their hegemonic control over the processes of healing actions carried out in intensive care.

Resistance

By contrast, critical moments of opposition that resist domination are liberating for people in that they are enabled to become

increasingly free to choose from a range of alternative perspectives on themselves and their social worlds. this freedom of choice requires the ability to see one's own view of what is good or right, possible or impossible, true or false, as problematic, socially constructed, and subject to social and political influence. (Berlak 1985:2)

This emancipatory activity by a subordinate group will, of necessity, meet with opposition from the dominant culture (Fay 1977). Giroux (1983:110) describes resistance as "an analytical construct and mode of inquiry that contains a moment of critique and a potential sensitivity to its own interests" of radical consciousness-raising and collective critical action. He argues that it is important to analyze all oppositional forms of behavior by making them a focal point for dialogue and critique to determine if they constitute a form of resistance. Williams (1977) reminds us that most alternative or oppositional forms are still tied to the dominant culture by virtue of their development in relation to the dominant ideology.

This is to argue that most forms of resistance are products of, and limited by, the dominant hegemony. Gender and nursing analyses that define themselves in opposition to patriarchal or medical cultures demonstrate this concept. However, analyses that develop a women-centered or nursing-centered ideology, which ignore male and/or medical domination, can provide an independent and original contribution representing an authentic alternative culture. This alternate culture can provide a paradigm that forces the dominant culture to accommodate to it. This is demonstrated in the development of areas of women's studies that focus on exploring women's knowledge and experiences in the face of critique that uses male-centered characteristics as standards of authority. Many of these courses are being incorporated into the dominant education systems. In this case the dominant ideology of scholarship has responded by incorporating the plethora of work produced by those women who challenged this ideology by ignoring it and developing their own criteria for authenticity, their own publishing houses, and their own strategies for sharing their work such as consciousness-raising groups and communal workshops (Spender 1981). These kinds of alternate analyses rather than oppositional analyses are rare but demonstrate the limits and pressures at work upon the ideological control represented in hegemony.

Nursing

Despite the generality of the term *nursing* I have chosen to use it in preference to the term *nursing profession,* which is becoming more popular in nursing scholarship. To support this decision I would like to briefly elaborate on the current debate on professional status as it relates to nursing before supplying a brief clarification of the term *nursing* as it is used in this thesis.

Theorists interested in describing the concept of professionalism and cataloging the professional status of various occupations conclude that nursing can only be classified as a semiprofession (Etzioni 1969; Friedson 1970). This categorization is based on the fact that many nurses work part time and don't have a high level of commitment to nursing, that nursing has not developed a recognizable unique body of knowledge and skill, that nurses do not have discretionary authority or autonomy and are not legitimated as professionals by community sanction. These analyses were carried out in the late 1960s but recent nursing analyses using these criteria have argued that nursing is still a semiprofession (Chapman 1977; Chaska 1978; Roberts 1980) or at an "emergent" stage (Tiffany 1982; Crowder 1985; Rogers 1985). These latter authors base their arguments on historical grounds by claiming that the recent advances in these areas suggest a changed status for nursing. These analyses share a common acceptance of these criteria of professionalism and the desirability of nursing being regarded as a profession. Chaska (1978) suggests that the public is increasingly skeptical about professions, but she uses this as the basis for her contention that nursing will need to work hard to achieve accountability within its drive for professional status.

The basis of professional status has been challenged and analyzed in other places (Illich 1977; Schön 1983). It has been suggested that professions are disabling by producing an uncritical, emotionally and economically dependant clientele. Oakley (1986) argues that the common criteria for professional status is male-created because the arguments about lack of commitment to employment and to long training programs is based on figures of the male-dominated "true" professions as against those for the female-dominated semiprofessions, where intervals out of the workforce for child rearing are considered evidence of lack of commitment. She suggests that nurses may like to question the value of being designated a profession if it means denying "at least half of humanity's needs and potential—the need and capacity for caring about oneself and others as whole people, not merely as sets of specialized and segmented skills" (Oakley 1986:193).

Some nurse leaders support the argument that professional characteristics are male-dominated but suggest that it is important for nursing to critique medical domination so that they can move towards professionalism (Ashley 1972; Melosh 1982; Speedy 1987). They contend that the aim of this move to professional status is for nursing to be recognized as independent of and equal to medicine in its contributions to healthcare and in receipt of parity in wages and conditions.

I would support this position for equity and parity, but I would like to shift the focus away from designations such as professional and semiprofessional. Autonomy in clinical nursing practice needs to be examined within a framework of responsibility for nursing actions and decisions, and in relation to patient advocacy and patient autonomy rather than in relation to medicine and its practices. An examination of medical domination is useful for an understanding of nursing oppression, but I would contend that this analysis should lead nurses away from a desire to emulate the dominators in the development of nursing. In this way nurses can begin to work together to critique the hegemony of the medical model and to begin to be accountable to themselves, their nursing peers, their patients, and their coworkers who may include doctors.

The term *nursing* then represents all those people who are registered to act as nurses and includes their knowledge, skills, and experience, whether informally present in practice or formally codified within nursing theories or education, in nursing research or union representation, in nursing administration, and in the diversities of nursing roles and practice settings. This definition is advantaged by being comprehensive but limited by its complexity. Therefore, I have chosen to designate nursing roles by their specific labels when appropriate— intensive care nurse, charge nurse, nurse educator, nurse researcher, psychiatric nurse—and nursing settings are treated similarly. The most common setting for nursing is still the hospital despite the number of openings for nurses in community, school, and industrial settings. Clinical nursing practice represents the setting of nurses who are engaged in nursing patients rather than engaging in other activities, which are part of the wider concept of nursing.

Critical theory

Critical theory is a term which is subject to different understandings and uses. Commonly it is a view of theory that has developed through the work done by members of the Institute for Social Research created in Frankfurt, Germany, in 1923 and known as the Frankfurt school. The members of the Frankfurt school critiqued the view that it is possible to apply the same paradigm and methodology used in the natural sciences, often labeled positivism, by disclosing the mechanisms of ideological control implicit in the consciousness and practices of advanced capitalist societies (Giroux 1983). They advocated a critique of society that challenges the basic social assumptions, which maintain cultural hegemony, and argued that the adoption of a technocratic view of science celebrated "facts" and stripped knowledge of its ethical and critical components by reducing it to the phenomena that is derived from the experience of the senses. This technocratic view suppressed the elements of subjectivity in knowledge, the capacity to develop a critical consciousness, and the influence of the elements of a sociocultural world. The members of the Frankfurt school argued that an examination of the elements of contradictions and domination in the social world is possible through the process of critical thinking that forms the basis for the kind of collaborative rational dialogue, which is a neces-

sary component in their struggles to transform their self-consciousness in order to effect social change.

Fay (1987:27) describes a critical theory as a theory that
wants to explain a social order in such a way that it becomes
itself the catalyst that leads to the transformation of this social
order. Carr and Kemmis (1983) suggest that a critical theory is
the product of an engagement in the process of critique that
transforms conscious ways of thinking without necessarily
changing practices in the world. Only when a critical theory is
combined with the political determination to act to empower
people to overcome the contradictions and oppression in their
daily lives does it become what Habermas described as critical
social science (Habermas 1971).

Critical social science

Fay (1975) states that a critical social science can be
characterized by three main features. The first feature is a
rejection of the positivist model of social science and an acceptance of the necessity of interpretive categories. He argues that
an understanding of how actors perceive their world is an
essential first step to the development of an authentic critique
of their social situation as a prelude towards emancipatory
change. The critical model asserts that in order to have a subject matter at all the social scientist must attempt to understand the intentions and desires of the actors he is observing,
as well as the rules and constitutive meanings of their social
order (Fay 1975:93–4).

However, unlike social scientists working from an interpretive paradigm, critical social scientists recognize the ideological
nature of these interpretations because they can be shaped by
distorted and unexamined views of reality. Fay (1975) describes
this process of enlightenment of the ideological nature of self-
understandings as the second feature of a critical social science. That is to say, a recognition that a great many of the
actions people perform are not the result of conscious knowledge and choice but are caused by social conditions over which
they have no control. Therefore, a critical social science endeavors to uncover "those systems of social relationships which
determine the actions of individuals and the unanticipated consequences of these actions" (Fay 1975:94).

In a different context, Freire (1972) describes the ideological blindness of people who have been oppressed—a distortion

of reality deriving from their "adherence" to the oppressor. The oppressed do not perceive themselves as the actors or subjects in their own social drama but as objects participating in the drama of the oppressors. One characteristic, exhibited by members of oppressed groups, is the tendency to secretly admire the behavior of the oppressor and to begin to imitate it. This implies a noncritical acceptance of the values and behavior exhibited by the oppressor. Fay (1977) states that it is not only important for people to come to a new self-understanding as the basis for altering social arrangements, but also important is the manner in which they come to adopt this new "guiding idea." He says that rational discourse must be the basis upon which the oppressed person makes a change in his basic self-conception. This process of rational discourse includes an acceptance of the place of historical accounts in an understanding of social situations and social conflict. Freire (1972) contrasts the notion of rational discourse or dialogue with the "banking model" in which the oppressed are seen as passive recipients of the information that the oppressors judge will be useful for them. Fay (1977) explains that the process of coming to a radical new self-conception hardly ever occurs simply by reading some theoretical work. Rather, he suggests,

> it requires an environment of trust, openness, and support in which one's own perceptions and feelings can be made properly conscious to oneself, in which one can think through one's experiences in terms of a radically new vocabulary which expresses a fundamentally different conceptualization of the world, in which one can see the particular and concrete ways that one unwittingly collaborates in producing one's own misery, and in which one can gain the emotional strength to accept and act on one's new insights. (Fay 1977:232)

What Fay is pointing to here is the essential interrelationship of theory and practice in critical social science, a concept elaborated by Habermas (1971). Freire (1972:29) writes of the reflection as the basis for an integration of theory and practice:

> But action is human only when it is not merely an occupation but also a preoccupation, that is, when it is not dichotomized from reflection.

This reflection faciltates enlightenment as a basis for liberatory or empowering practices, which may combine to bring
about emancipation. Therefore, critical social science can be
recognized as a process with a specific interest in the elements
of enlightenment, empowerment, and emancipation (Fay 1987).

Critical pedagogy

Discourses are formed historically and ideologically to
represent, through language and practices, the meanings,
actions, and identities of cultural groups. Critical pedagogy is
not a familiar concept to many nurse educators; rather, in
many circles, it has been understood as a term that describes
strategies and techniques designed to meet classroom teaching
goals. Indeed, the interest in the strategies and principles of
adult education has influenced many nurse educators to rele-
gate the term *pedagogy* to the realm of the classroom education of children.

I believe that nursing needs to appropriate the insights of
critical pedagogy, not only as a means of informing and shaping nursing curricula practices but as a means of understanding and shaping the nursing role in the interests of empowering healthcare. The provision of enabling and empowering
healthcare requires an understanding of the repressive myths
of the cultural sites in which healthcare is practiced and provided and the processes to develop more enlightened and liberating practices.

As Simon suggests:

if we want to examine how our practice relates to future
visions of community life we need to provide an alternative to the impoverishing constriction imposed by an
exclusive reliance on practical suggestions and the reduc-
tion of the debate to questions of "what works." The discourse of pedagogy provides such an alternative. (1988:2)

What then are the principle components of a discourse of
pedagogy? For nurses, the instigation of a modern understanding of a relationship between pedagogy, language, culture, and
liberatory politics can perhaps be traced to the seminal work of
Paulo Freire in *Pedagogy of the Oppressed* (1972). Freire's interest in articulating and changing the experiences of oppressed
people resonates with many nurses who have experienced the

double oppression of medical domination and patriarchy. For Freire culture is always a multidimensional structural formation representing historic, economic, class, and political relations reflected in language. He argues for an understanding of culture as a field of struggle where a language of critique and a language of hope are formed and lived (Freire 1985).

Simon argues for an understanding of critical pedagogy that is concerned with pedagogical practice as a project of possibility. This project requires a "view of human freedom as the *understanding of necessity and the transformation of necessity*" (Simon 1988:2, original emphasis). According to Simon, although much of the work of critical pedagogy has been located in schools, it is important to recognize that pedagogy reflects any practice that intentionally tries to influence the production of cultural meaning. The nursing role is enacted in a variety of community and institutional sites where nurses are engaged in the processes of making meaning of patterns and experiences of health and illness for themselves and their patients/clients. An engagement in critical pedagogy enables nurses to deconstruct the ideological, political, and historical elements of nursing discourse and to use metaphoric imagination to reconstruct a collaborative social dream of transformative healthcare, which is reflected in a transformative discourse of healing. This discourse would take account of the fragility of points of accomodation and resistance in nursing practice in order to develop alternative discourses and action that challenge and resist the dominant discourses of medicine and nursing. McLaren (1989:242) contends that:

> Critical discourse must call for a new narrative through which a qualitatively better world can be both imagined and struggled for. We must be united in the face of overwhelming odds, and the pedagogy we use must be capable of inflating the human capacity to vie with forces of domination at a scale that makes us reject despair and refuse capitulation to the status quo.

This is the project of critical pedagogy, a project that nurses are beginning to actively address in the literature and the nursing curricula and a project that needs attention at the sites of cultural struggle, the world of clinical practice.

7

❦

Charting the Theoretical Terrain

A knowledge of the nature of the terrain is important in any journey of discovery. It provides the intrepid traveler with the necessary information by which to make sense of the territory to be traveled. This helps the traveler make the necessary preparations in order to be able to traverse the territory effectively and in a way that meets the traveler's goals. This journey of discovery was to be taken using a map created from the theoretical structures of the literature of the feminist and critical traditions of thought. By choosing this map I was identifying the theoretical signposts that would be aiding me in my travels. Key signposts were the concepts of enlightenment, empowerment, emancipation, and power/knowledge.

Action: Embedded, Informed, and Transformed by Technical, Practical, and Emancipatory Knowledge

Nursing actions are dialectically related to nursing knowledge. This dialectic relationship represents the continual interchange between the practices engaged in by nurses and the particular forms of knowledge in which these practices are embedded and by which they are informed and transformed. The synthesis of this dialectic, within an isolated and contextually dependent situation in the sociocultural world of nursing practice, creates a new dialectic between the changed action and the changed knowledge held by the nurse practitioner. The forms of knowledge used by nurses engaged in nursing practice can be differentiated by the human interests that they serve. Jurgen Habermas (1971) argues that it is not possible to provide an objective or neutral account of reality because contending human interests develop knowledge through processes that cannot be described as pure, objective, or disinterested. Rather, there is more than one kind of valid knowledge because knowledge is shaped within the context of social, historical, and cultural conditions and is determined by specific needs desires and interests. Habermas designated his theory of competing knowledge claims a theory of "knowledge-constitutive interests" and argued that these interests are *a priori* because they precede the act of cognition by constituting the mode of thought prior to the thought processes. The knowledge-constitutive interests frame the cognitive processes, which develop the construction of reality.

Habermas developed this theory in order to place techni-cal reason within a comprehensive theory of rationality. He argued that this comprehensive concept of reason had been reduced to *scientism*, which is a reliance upon and acceptance of the exclusive validity of scientific and technical thought. In other words valid knowledge had been reduced to science's belief in itself. This scientism conceals the transcendental basis of facts and descriptions in which meaning is generated from structures of experience and action, through critical, philosophical inquiry and reflection. Accordingly, scientism protects scientific inquiry from epistemology, the theory of the basis and grounds for knowledge. Habermas argues that this objectifying process has led to the abandonment of stages of reflection by which the subject can examine and critique the relationship between knowledge and human interests.

Unlike his predecessors Horkheimer, Marcuse, and Adorno in the German Institute of Social Research, Habermas argued that the problem lay not with technical reason, as such, but with its exclusiveness and universality for the devel-opment of valid knowledge. He agreed with their contentions that science had become an ideology that legitimated social action by the production of objective facts thereby stripping knowledge of its ethical and critical components, but he was not prepared to replace technical rationality with the philo-sophical dimension of critical reasoning. He declared that tech-nical knowledge was valuable for humanity and, as such, was a necessary form of knowledge that served a human interest in control over the natural world. However, he argued that other forms of knowledge were equally valid and necessary for humanity. Habermas went on to categorize three competing forms of knowledge-constitutive interests—the *technical*, the *practical*, and the *emancipatory*.

The technical interest is concerned with causal explanations in which instrumental knowledge facilitates technical control over natural objects. Action is directed to technical mastery, produces nomological knowledge and is described as "instrumental action." The development of technical knowledge requires a disinterested attitude to the object of inquiry. The technical interest is mediated in the sociocultural sphere of work and reproduction, and is the domain of the empirical-analytic or natural sciences. This domain produces the knowledge necessary for the processes of industry and production along with biophysical basis of medicine and nursing and the medical technology that supports and incorporates this knowledge. Habermas affirms the place of technical knowledge but argues that many aspects of sociocultural life are symbolically structured and cannot be represented by instrumental knowledge.

According to Habermas, specific methodological procedures, such as the *verstehen* methods of the hermeneutic tradition, which seek to develop theoretical interpretations to disclose the subjective meanings of action, are necessary to reveal reliable intersubjectivity in ordinary language communication. This emphasis on reciprocity in understanding, as in *verstehen*, is the focus of practical knowledge, which informs and guides practical wisdom and judgement. This practical action produces nomological knowledge and is directed to reciprocity in symbolic interactions mediated by language and described as "communicative action."

Habermas regards the practical knowledge, which is based on communicative action, as valuable for the explications of subjective meanings but he argues that it fails to account for the objective context, which shapes and limits the subject's intentions and their realization. This suggests that communicative action may represent an unreflected consciousness, which is unable to assess the distortion and repression caused by the sociocultural or political context.

As a response to this critique Habermas elaborated a third form of knowledge, which serves the human interest in freedom, rationality, and autonomy and which he called emancipatory knowledge. This emancipatory knowledge is guided by

critical theory, which recognizes its explicit intent to inform
and transform the self-understandings of people so that they
can collaboratively engage in transformative actions. Habermas was indebted to the work of Marx in the development of
ideology as a critique of political economy (Habermas 1973a).
However, he went on to argue that the advent of advanced capitalism meant that politics should not be only regarded as a
phenomena of the superstructure because this view allowed
practical issues to be defined as technical problems making
the role of the public sphere one of choosing between alternative groups of administrators and technicians. This choice
denies humanity's interest in emancipation because it serves
the interest of a particular group. When politics is recognized
as also operating at a micro level within practical issues, then
critique can focus attention on the oppressive forms of sociocultural life and on the modes of thinking that re-create and
maintain this hegemony.

According to Habermas, emancipatory knowledge locates
ideological distortion and repression through the process of self-
reflection, which has two dimensions. McCarthy (1985) suggests that the first dimension relates to a critique of knowledge
when self-reflection means reflection on the subjective conditions of knowledge within the normative objective context of
facts. He describes the second dimension as a critique of ideology in which self-reflection reveals the dialectic of repressed processes and language, which constitute a distorted worldview.
The emancipatory interest of self-reflection guides the rational
pursuit of goals. Action is directed to individual and collaborative enlightenment as the basis for empowerment and social
transformation. This transformative action is the process of
emancipation and the development of emancipatory knowledge.

Habermas (1971) recognizes the tentative and exploratory
nature of the exposition of this view of a human interest in
emancipatory knowledge. He is engaged in a process of continually redeveloping and redefining his theory in response to his
numerous critics, some of whom are supportive of the theory of
knowledge-constitutive interests but have difficulties with its
explication.

An early and important criticism was the charge of elitism
(McCarthy 1985). It was suggested that critical theorists were
able to employ their own normative prejudices under the guise
of rationality by which to make judgements on the "true" inter-

pretations of life. In response Habermas (1971) evolved his theory of communicative competence, a theory that Carr and Kemmis (1983:139) describe as an "ethical theory of self-realization which transposes the source of human ideals onto language and discourse." Essentially this is an argument for a form of discourse which facilitates a cooperative search for truth leading to the development of rational autonomy. Habermas (1971) argues that discourse discloses the truth claims of opinions, which are no longer taken for granted by the speakers. In discourse four validity claims are used in order that, through the structuring of rational argument based on these validity claims, a true and appropriate consensus can be established. The validity claims require that what is stated is true, comprehensible, spoken in sincerity by the speaker, and that the speaker has a right to be engaging in the speech act. According to Habermas, when these conditions are met then true dialogue can ensue with the potential for developing emancipatory knowledge. Therefore, an understanding of Habermas' concept of discourse is integral to an understanding of the process by which knowledge is constituted with an emancipatory interest.

Fraser (1987) contends that feminist studies have found that the capacities for consent and speech in public debate are connected with masculinity in a patriarchal advanced capitalism. She argues that there is a "conceptual dissonance between femininity and the dialogical capacities central to Habermas's conception of citizenship" (Fraser 1987:44). The pairing of reason with critical self-reflection led to the charge that Habermas was jeopardizing the claim of reason to universality. Questions were raised concerning the status of knowledge-constitutive interests. Were they merely contingent empirical interests, social products subject to change, or transcendental interests, which are fundamental and beyond historical confines?

In reworking his position to elucidate his framework more clearly, Habermas (1973b) moved away from his earlier adaptation of themes from classical German thought and redefined his concept of "critical self-reflection" by replacing it with "rational reconstruction." This redefinition shifted the emphasis from a reliance on a process of self-critique and reflection, putting more emphasis on the development of ideal speech situations as the basis for critique. By pursuing this changed emphasis, which arguably reopens the theory/practice gap, Habermas laid himself open to what is probably the most important criticism of his concept of critical theory. It has been charged that critical theory, with its ideological basis of emancipatory knowledge with a practical intent, remains an ideal rather than a reality and that its protagonists are engaging in rhetoric that is not grounded in practice. Fay (1987) alleges that it is necessary for people to engage in critical social science in order that their self-reflection can lead them to a recognition of the conditions necessary for the development of emancipatory knowledge and of the dialectic at work in the sociocultural world that limits and constrains transformative action.

A critical social science that ignores the place of technical and practical knowledge in nursing practice will in itself represent distortion and repression. However, an examination of nursing practice that recognizes the technical and practical knowledge necessary in the discipline of nursing can take up the challenge to develop emancipatory knowledge in and through the process of critique, reflection, and transformative action.

Technical knowledge in clinical nursing practice enables nurses to understand and predict the biophysical behavior of their patients and to use this knowledge in the interface with medical technological interventions. An understanding of the causal explanations of biophysical, chemical, psychological, and sensory-motor reactions in the systems of the body is essential for the development of skilled nurses able to assess and plan appropriate instrumental action. This use of technical knowledge in nursing has been documented extensively and will not be challenged here. What is being challenged is the totality of a worldview in which technical knowledge is accepted as *the* normative knowledge by which nursing is constituted and understood.

Communicative Action: Reclaiming the Meanings

Practical knowledge in clinical nursing practice informs and guides practical judgement. This judgement is essential to enlighten nurses about the ways in which technical interventions affect the lives of patients and others participating in the sociocultural world of nursing practice. Symbolic interactions between nurse and patient, nurse and nurse, nurse and allied health workers, nurse and significant others in the lives of their patients are mediated through the language processes of communicative action.

A commitment to the development of practical knowledge through language prompted Gadamer (1975) to challenge Habermas's (1971) development of an emancipatory human interest by enlarging on his own description of the *verstehen* method of articulating language meanings. Held (1980:312) describes Gadamer's understanding of *verstehen* as an "'effective–historical consciousness' constituted by a language community." This concept is used in relation to the concept of tradition, which for Gadamer (1975) is a total cultural background containing practices, vocabulary, concepts, and hypotheses, all of which he characterizes as preunderstanding—the prejudices and prejudgements that condition the process of understanding. He argues that understanding is integrally linked to interpretation. According to Gadamer, the interpreters bring to the interpretations their own norms, beliefs, practices, and concepts, all of the expectations that have developed from their worldview. He declares that this subjective nature of interpretation is crucial to the development of meaning. He argues that language and tradition are interrelated and that the process of human understanding is a process of discovering inherited biases and prejudgements in dialogue with others. Gadamer claims that through the linguistic experiences of shared dialogue both prejudices and prejudgements are able to be judged as enabling or as blind.

This kind of practical knowledge is essential for nurses who need to develop reciprocal communications with patients, and others, based on mutual understandings of the symbolic nature of the nursing context and its historical construction. Nurses need to engage in shared dialogue to uncover biases and prejudices, which influence their interpretations of the nursing situation. Nurse scholars have become increasingly aware of the value of practical knowledge, and accordingly the interpretive paradigm has gained credibility and inclusion in most Australian nursing curricula. This approach does not seriously challenge the supremacy of the positivist paradigm within nursing with its emphasis on technical knowledge based on instrumental reason. However, nurses are increasingly interested in incorporating practical knowledge with technical knowledge in order to describe and understand nursing actions within a framework of intersubjective meanings and nursing tradition. Although this knowledge is useful and necessary to nursing, it does not allow for the ways in which tradi-

tion and communicative action can conceal and distort as well
as reveal and express (McCarthy 1985). Nor does it account for
the false consciousness that may be reflected in agreed upon
intersubjective meanings.

In developing a response to Gadamer, Habermas (1973b)
stressed that language is not only related to tradition but is also
a medium for domination and social power. He argued that language can be used for deception as easily as for interpretation.
Therefore, it becomes necessary to engage in reflection in order
to reveal hidden meanings and then to critique them. The basis
of Habermas's (1971) contention is that hermeneutics does not
make ideological relations explicit and so it is possible to develop a functionalist position from the subjective determining of a
hermeneutic perspective. Thompson (1985), Allen (1985), and
Perry (1986) acknowledge the value of Habermas's work for the
development of nursing. They argue that emancipatory knowledge is necessary to generate a critique of the repression and
distortion inherent in clinical nursing practice. The medium of
this emancipatory knowledge is power and the process in which
it engages is the process of reflection.

Reflection: Confrontation and Reconstruction

Habermas (1971) used Marx's ideology critique and
Freudian psychoanalysis in his development of an appropriate
methodology for the growth of enlightenment and emancipatory
knowledge. He asserted that an unreflected, natural consciousness is a false consciousness, which is bound in dogmatism
and error. The key to "intuition and emancipation, comprehension and liberation from dogmatic dependence" is found in the
process of self-reflection (Habermas 1973b:156). Using Freud's
concept of the process of psychoanalysis, Habermas argues for
a methodology of self-reflection that brings the unconscious,
taken-for-granted, habitual ways of thinking and reasoning to
the surface for ideology critique and reconstruction in such a
manner that the cognitive processes and the self-formative processes merge. In this merger Habermas alleges that knowledge
and action are fused into a single entity.

According to Freire (1981), human beings are active agents
who are capable of reflecting on themselves, on the activity in
which they are engaged, and on the social world in which they
live. He suggests that through this process of self-reflection and

collaborative rational discourse, human beings are able to penetrate the hegemonic structures that support oppression and discover the true interrelationships between facts. In this process of collaboration and reciprocity, thought, action, and reflection combine in informed committed action—a praxis—to develop a critical enlightenment. Fay (1977) states that critical enlightenment leads to liberation when people understand the ways in which they have become implicated in the causes of social repression and are then able to take committed, concerted action to bring about social change. Reflection facilitates the development of self-determination by enabling people who had functioned as objects in the world, to transform themselves into active subjects. This emancipatory process of reflection enables the subject to confront and reconstruct knowledge and action. Therefore, reflection can be recognized as a counterhegemonic process.

Giroux (1983) builds on these ideas by underscoring the importance of neo-Marxist notions of resistance and reproduction in the reflective process of emancipation. Reproduction theories focus on the manner in which power is used to support the interests of the dominant groups in society (Anyon 1984). These theories are concerned with the reproduction of the social relations and attitudes that sustain the interests of capital. Reproduction theories are useful in their challenges to value-free knowledge and objective actions but are limited by their lack of acknowledgement of the areas of daily life that cannot be described in relation to a capitalist ideology (Giroux 1983). Their neglect of oppositional moments of resistance, and of a focus on radical social change, means that reproduction theories can become deterministic and negative.

By contrast theories of resistance provide a study of the way in which class and culture combine to offer outlines for a cultural politics (Giroux 1983). This cultural politics enables the analysis of counterhegemonic elements in the cultural field of the oppressed, which includes the elements of style, rituals, language, and systems of meaning. Freire (1985) reminds us that counterhegemonic elements can be stripped of their radical power for social change by adaption and incorporation into the dominant culture. Giroux (1983) argues that resistance theories can reveal and critique domination through the provision of theoretical opportunities for self-reflection. This reflexive process is developed through a number of analyses that point to those nonreproductive "moments" that constitute and support the critical notion of human agency. Theories of resistance develop forms of political analyses that have the power to study and transform radical themes, and those social practices that make up the class-based cultural fields and details of everyday life, including the sociocultural world of clinical nursing practice. This requires critical analyses of the language of nursing in order to reveal oppressive attitudes and actions. McLaren (1988a:3) reminds us that language cannot be "conceptualized as a transparent window to the world but rather constitutes a symbolic medium that actively shapes and transforms the word." Here McLaren is alerting us to the ideological component of language the fact that language is

> always situated within ideology and power/knowledge relations that govern and regulate access particular interpretive communities have to language practices. (McLaren 1988a:3)

Therefore, language is situated within discourses, which are subject to the interpretation and legitimation of the dominant cultural group. Nursing language reflects both the influence of the dominant discourse of medicine and the unacknowledged traditions and assumptions that have shaped and formed nursing as subordinate to medicine. Comments such as "only a nurse," "she's a born nurse," "I am not a theoretical nurse just a good practical nurse," and "nurses are their own worst enemies" demonstrate the effects of the legitimation of medical knowledge over nursing knowledge. It is difficult to imagine that the preceding comments could have been uttered by medical staff about themselves; the comment "only a doctor" is inconsistent with the socially legitimated status acceded to medical staff. For resistance to occur means that nursing staff need to support each other to undo oppressive language practices and to support and re-create liberating discourse.

Bullough (1984) argues that a focus on resistance, as opposition to authority or control, is inadequate without an understanding of the nature of the role of the subject. He contends that role is taken-for-granted and ideologically embedded, and an analysis of role is necessary to uncover the history of structural constraints, the potential and constraints upon human interaction and the development of consciousness. This emphasis allows resistance to be recognized as those actions that challenge role boundaries, thereby making possible the distinction between acts with radical potential and those without. Bullough argues that this focus allows for an understanding of resistance as being comprised of two moments—those that confront internalized limitations and those that challenge the external, institutional structures.

The relationship between role and resistance is a valuable concept in an analysis of nursing practice. Reflection on the role of the clinical nurse and on those actions of resistance that challenge role boundaries facilitates the discovery of emancipatory knowledge for nursing.

A further examination of the relationship between resistance and knowledge occurs at the point where knowledge ceases and ignorance begins. McLaren (1988a), using the work of Shoshana Felman on Jacques Lacan (1987), articulates this most eloquently when he writes:

> Ignorance is part of the very structure of knowledge—the part that escapes intentionality and meaning. Ignorance is that which is not remembered—which refuses to be remembered; it is what is repressed or actively excluded from consciousness: What we won't admit to knowledge. It is, in effect, a desire to ignore the will to forget. *Ignorance is situated at the point knowledge is resisted* (1988a:7, my emphasis).

McLaren extends this analysis to expose the subjugation of different "voices" representing diverse alternative discourses, which have been repressed by the intensity of the dominant discourse. Ignorance of the content of these marginalized voices enables processes of hegemonic domination to be maintained and the cries of resistance to be silenced.

Knowledge-Constitutive Interests and Power/Knowledge

The search for these silenced and domesticated forms of knowledge is a search for emancipatory knowledge—a form of knowledge that Habermas (1971) contended is constituted by a specific cognitive interest in rational autonomy. This search for emancipatory knowledge is based on the assumption that through the process of reflection and rational analysis people can understand themselves, their histories and the mechanisms by which they collude in their own oppression, and by knowing, can change themselves and their situation. This process is based on the premise that enlightenment enables people to empower themselves.

A concern with this argument revolves around the question of whether knowledge-constitutive interests are contingent or transcendental. A French philosopher, Michel Foucault (1982), took the position that Habermas's interests in finalized activity and capacity (technical knowledge), communication (practical knowledge), and domination or power (emancipatory knowledge) were not separate domains of knowledge but overarching transcendentals. Foucault challenged the notion that these are, in reality, knowledge-constitutive interests; he contended that these are in fact types of relationships which overlap, reciprocally support, and mutually use each other. He alleges that domination is found in each of these interrelated interests in different forms. These relationships of domination are not uniform or constant; they establish themselves in different forms in different circumstances, and these varying interrelationships constitute a particular "model" for a particular context. Foucault argues that the shape of these models are determined by "blocks." These blocks relate to form a framework composed of regulated and concerted systems through which the operationalizing of technical capacities, the activities of communication, and the relationships of power interrelate and adjust. These systems of relationships give different emphasis to power relations depending on the institutional framework in which it is constituted, in Foucault's terms, its "disciplines." Foucault examines disciplines such as hospitals, prisons, and apprenticeships in order to demonstrate the different emphases of power relationships operating within the structures.

This concept of power relationships challenges the empirical notion of a formal, theoretical, and united scientific discourse by advocating the development of discourses based on differential, local knowledges, which will of necessity be fragmented and discontinuous. Foucault (1982) suggests that the activity of developing these forms of discourse puts them immediately at risk of cooption by the power relations that they set out to challenge. The knowledge uncovered by these discourses is cataloged, accredited, and used in ways which

enable them to become recodified within the prevailing dominant discourse.

By reworking Habermas's concept of knowledge-constitutive interests, Foucault establishes a discourse that shifts the
focus of an examination of power from questions of what power
is and where it comes from to an examination of power relations through the question "How is power exercised?" By posing this question Foucault (1975) contends that an analysis
that identifies power as the medium in which emancipatory
knowledge is generated, separates power from knowledge. He
asserts that knowledge and power are inseparable and interrelated, that they directly imply one another, that there is no
power relation without the correlative constitution of a field of
knowledge nor any knowledge that does not presuppose and
constitute at the same time power relations.

Foucault states that the analysis of power/knowledge relations consists of processes and struggles of power/knowledge,
which determine the forms and possible domains of knowledge.
This challenges the view that an engagement in an activity such
as reflection or rational argument enables the subject to develop knowledge that is resistant to power. According to Foucault,
this is a negative view in which power and knowledge are external to each other with knowledge being related to truth and
power being equated with oppression and repression. Foucault
(1980b:84) labels this view of power the "juridico-discursive"
and alleges that this view of power has been accepted into discourse for two historically based reasons.

The first reason for the development of the juridico-discursive view is the separation of power and truth for the
"speaker's benefit." Discussion on a hitherto repressed topic
places the speaker outside the reach of power. The speaker can
then solemnly appeal to the future in a prophetic voice as the
harbinger of truth. This promise of a brighter, better world
enables the speaker to adopt a privileged position from which
to judge present oppression against the promises of the new
order. This is the role of the universal intellectual, perhaps the
critical theorist, who in the role of prophet and judge is exempt
from charges of involvement in repression.

The second reason for the acceptance of this view of power
as oppression and repression is the unrecognized relationship
between power and knowledge. This relationship is masked by
the production of a discourse designed to locate power as a

"pure limit set on freedom" (Foucault 1980b:86). Foucault
argues that this pre-occupation with power as limit and repression is deceptive because it disguises the power/knowledge
relationship by locating it within a discourse on power. Foucault
claims that the discourse that locates power as limit and repression is in itself part of an exercise of modern power/knowledge.

Foucault describes this legitimation of a schism between
power and knowledge as a repressive hypothesis and argues
that this enables power to hide its own mechanisms. For Foucault emancipatory knowledge must always be power/knowl-
edge; the knowledge that is exposed when the question of how
power is exercised is addressed. This power/knowledge proceeds from power relationships, which Foucault defines as a
mode of action that does not act directly and immediately on
others.

> Instead it acts upon their actions: an action upon an
> action, on existing actions or on those which may arise in
> the present or the future. (1982:220)

Foucault alleges that this set of actions acting upon other
actions can be brought about by violence or consensus, by
acceptance or seduction, by induction or inciting, but the end
result is always action upon the action of others. The manner
by which these power relations can be analyzed is by focusing
on carefully circumscribed institutions.

This process immediately meets with problems. Institutions such as hospitals maintain their existence by a series of
mechanisms, which are productive and reproductive in function but which serve to mask the power relations at work. Analyzing power relations from an institutional framework pre-
sents the risk of explaining the relationships in the light of that
framework. Foucault argues that this risk comes from an
apparatus or *dispositif,* by which he means the use of concepts
as tools, being put into contention against explicit and implicit
regulations so that the power relations are reduced to descriptions of legalism and coercion.

An examination of power relations which can lead us to
an explication of power/knowledge requires that a number of
points be addressed. Foucault (1982:223) begins this process
with what he describes as the "system of differentiations." This
enables the analysis to locate those knowledge differences that

enable one party to act upon another because of their privileged access to economic, linguistic, cultural, or social know-how, skills, or competence. The system of differentiations within healthcare would reveal the differences in access to socially legitimated knowledge, skills, and practices that doctors enjoy over all other members of the healthcare team. From this Foucault moves to an examination of the "types of objectives" such as profit or status, which are pursued by those who act upon the actions of others. The economic, cultural, and social objectives of doctors in relation to nurses and paramedics would be examined. Analysis of "the means of bringing power relations into being" reveals the mechanisms such as surveillance systems, threats of violence, or dismissal by which these objectives are achieved. Hospital administration, government health department, and senior medical and nursing staff collude formally and informally in the production and maintenance of mechanisms that develop power relations in healthcare settings. It is necessary to pursue the "forms of institutionalization" that support these mechanisms such as the traditional, legalized institutional form of the hospital with its clearly delineated hierarchical structures, regulations, and multiple apparatuses operating interrelatedly. The final point to be addressed is the "degree of rationalization" required to elaborate, transform, and organize these power relations in terms such as technological inputs and refinements or economic arguments pitting costs against eventual profits. Rationalizations abound in healthcare settings where arguments can be mounted to rationalize activities such as the cost of high technology useful for very few patients by pitting it against the emotional appeal of saving a life (it could be yours or the life of your loved one).

This process provides a useful framework for the analysis of sociocultural power relationships as a basis for revealing power/knowledge. However, it is interesting to note that Foucault did not take up the challenge to engage in a power/knowledge analysis as the basis for an engagement in emancipatory action. Despite Foucault's (1982) charges against the "negative" nature of the juridico-discursive view of power, his own analyses, which are concerned with "writing the history of the present," portray a negative present world. Unlike the promises of a better world offered by an engagement with emancipatory knowledge, Foucault's power/knowledge unmasks the current situation without providing any utopian hopes. Dreyfus (1982:109) in his charting of Foucault's work comments:

> Subjection, domination and combat are found everywhere he looks. Whenever he hears talk of meaning and value of virtue and goodness he looks for strategies of domination.

Foucault (1980b:143) contends that power/knowledge has in fact become "an agent for transformation of human life," but he sees this as a collective potentiality and denies the possibility of individual subjects being able to take control of their own lives. His emphasis on the need to uncover the power relations and the contention that this process can in itself create power relations means that the methodologies he used are not empowering methodologies based on action, reflection, and reconstructed action. He constructs his form of ideology critique in unique ways. His early work was based on archeological methodology but he became dissatisfied with the limitations of this method and moved on to develop genealogies. Genealogies allow Foucault the opportunity to take the role of diagnostician who focuses on power/knowledge and the body in modern society. This genealogical method is supported by a search for discontinuities and shifts in meaning characteristic of his earlier archeological method. Balbus (1987) challenges Foucault's concept of discontinuities because he contends that beneath the apparent discontinuities present in transitory historical forms is the hegemonic continuity of male domination. He suggests that it is possible to speak of a patriarchal historical continuity of Western thought, which, once recognized, is more pervasive than the transitory discontinuities. Balbas develops this idea by suggesting that the will to power/knowledge is treated by Foucault as gender-neutral, and so Foucault translates what is essentially a male orientation into a generically human orientation obliterating the distinctively female power of nurturance. Therefore, he argues that Foucault has a historical continuity with his own history of discontinuity through a focus on the will to power/knowledge.

In the context of his genealogy Foucault (1982) regards his role as that of diagnostician enabling him to locate and describe power relations at work, in particular disciplines. He describes the role of diagnostician as a specific intellectual role rather than a universal role as is subscribed to in his critique of the relations that operate to the speaker's benefit. However, he does not appear to identify the similarity of the power relations at work in the diagnostic role with those in the role that he rejects as the speaker's benefit.

Foucault repudiates the active subject who is the focus for critical social scientists because he contends that the subject is an effect of power/knowledge, and it is necessary to reject that subject to reveal the power/knowledge mechanism. However, this contrasts with Foucault's own role as diagnostician, the role of a subjective interpreter who constitutes and enacts the process. In effect this role can then become invisible rather than left open to contestation and critique. Balbas (1987:122) describes the role of diagnostician as "an animating source of the deconstructive discourse" suggesting that this emphasis reclaims the subjective role for the theorist/diagnostician.

In developing a framework in which to develop emancipatory power/knowledge that includes oppression, resistance, and nurturance, it is useful to examine Fay's recent work (1987). Fay's earlier work (1975) was based on Habermas's conception of a critical social science and in it Fay developed the argument that human beings are active beings capable of rationally reflecting on their lives and using this rational reflection as a basis for transformative action. This position assumed that it was possible for people to engage equally in rational discourse, a position that has been greatly challenged by feminists (Fraser 1987).

Spender (1981) argues that in sex-segregated groups, women develop cooperative mechanisms for discourse, many of which are nurturant and nonverbal. These skills would not be addressed by Habermas's guidelines for rational discourse because his theory is based on a generic orientation in which women are invisible and are then included in an essentially male orientation to the development of reciprocity in dialogue.

In response to gender critiques of the mechanisms of rational discourse and in response to Foucault's work on the relationship between discourse and embodiment, Fay (1987) suggests that his earlier position, which alleged that the capacity to engage in rational autonomy is necessary for the development of emancipation, is limited in two ways. The first kind of limit is essentially practical. It represents the recognition that human beings are not only active beings capable of reflecting on their situation but also embodied, historical, traditional, and embedded creatures. These practicalities of humanity limit the capacity for human beings to change in response to reason and enlightenment.

Fay's second concern is with the integrity of the ideal of rational autonomy, which is based on assumptions that individuals are capable of clarity, of becoming transparent to themselves and others as a basis for rationality, and that all members of a group will form a consensus if the material is handled rationally. He argues that tradition, personal history, and embeddedness in a network of causal relations limit the capacity of individuals and groups to reason with clarity and also to be able to agree to act upon that reasoning. Fay is also concerned that the kind of rational autonomy that might develop from this kind of engagement could be in opposition to the enhancement of happiness, and in fact might bring disatisfaction, by being in conflict with the individual's cultural tradition, which has shaped the way in which their desires are formed and materialized. I would suggest that this would particularly be the case when rational autonomy is formed in a male-dominated context such as healthcare, and it conflicts with the embedded female values and experiences that nurses bring to caring. This embeddedness in tradition conflicts with the concept that individuals may freely choose from a variety of options, which can be examined as if the individual is divorced from their culture and the specific situation.

In Fay's specification of embodiment as a limit to rational change, he intersects with Foucault's (1980b) work on the political technology of the body. Essentially the argument recognizes that human beings are not disembodied rational beings but are beings with a body that is subject to needs, direction, manipulation, force, and meticulous rituals, all of which impinge on the human's capacity for acting rationally and autonomously. Foucault's concept of a technology of the body as the localization of power/knowledge developed as an alternative to the juridico-discursive concept of power. As we have seen Foucault regards Habermas's knowledge-constitutive interests as representative of transcendental categories rather than as the basis of a model for transformative action. Foucault (1980:28) argues for a "body politic,"

> a set of material elements and techniques that serve as weapons, relays communication routes and supports for the power and knowledge relations that invest human

bodies and subjugate them by turning them into objects of knowledge.

Foucault not only demonstrates the basis for a body politic but highlights his repudiation of the primacy of the subject, a theme in the work of Habermas and his followers, in favor of a process of objectivizing the subject through what he calls "dividing practices." Through a process of division from others or through division within themselves, subjects become objects. Illness divides a person from the healthy population, and this process turns the person into an object for attention—one who is sick. Foucault's work in the "History of Sexuality" (1980b) was intended to demonstrate the way in which people develop the capacity to recognize themselves as subjects of sexuality. He suggests that an understanding of the objectivication of the subject is basic to an understanding of the strategies of power relations as expressed in human bodies. Foucault's concept of "bio-power" is concerned with the regulation of the processes of human regeneration and with "disciplinary power," which describes the mechanisms by which a subject is turned into an object to be manipulated. This disciplinary power provides a docile workforce, which not only responds to the wishes of others but responds with speed, efficiency, and technical mastery. This docility is produced by the disciplines, which are the mechanics of power. These disciplines are represented at a micro level where individual movements, gestures, and attitudes are coerced in very subtle ways. The object of control is the internal organization, the efficiency and economy of movements. The modality of control is continuous supervision of the process of the activity rather than of the result. These mechanics codify movements within time and space to produce docile bodies, which are utilitarian and obedient. The hospital contains a multiplicity of processes, which combine to produce docility in the patients, the staff, and visitors. These processes are not the result of a decision by people in a position of power to construct an apparatus of domination. Rather, they are the result of a long history of individual and often seemingly unimportant responses to needs and crises, which, when integrated and combined, form disciplinary power/knowledge relationships. The scale of these responses is often small and seemingly independent of other activities. The bodies of nurses are trained to make beds in a

regulated way that ensures efficiency and economy of movement and produces a disciplined result. Continuous supervision during training ensures that this process enables the
body of the nurse to become obedient to the dictum that the
bed must be made in a regulated, utilitarian, and disciplined
manner. Not only does the body of the nurse learn to obey and
automatically make a bed in the manner prescribed, but it also
learns to carry out this action within a particular time frame
and within a particular limited space.

Foucault argues that this disciplinary power achieves its
power/knowledge over the body through a web of interrelated
techniques. The disciplines use time and space to control the
limits that the body is able to challenge. Enclosure within an
institution in which the necessities for life are provided—meals,
beds, retail outlets, centers for leisure, relaxation, and exercise—restrict the prospective mobility of the body. In enclosed
institutions where the extent of the mobility of the individual
can be totally circumscribed through negative disincentives
such as out-of-bounds areas, time-limited breaks, and distance
from alternative outlets for necessities and through positive
incentives such as low-cost or free meals and proximity to other
necessities, the body is encouraged to remain within the enclosure during working hours. However, the disciplinary mechanism of space is not limited to a principle of enclosure; it works
in a flexible detailed manner according to the locality. Individuals are partitioned off into small spaces with limits to mobility
through task, status, and role. Individuals are then collected
into small groups of like skills and knowledge to establish presence and absence, supervision and surveillance, communications and interruptions. This knowledge enables utility in function and mastery in control. All space is codified with a function
so that individuals entering that space learn to act in predetermined ways while there. This use of space intersects with rank
and status so that individuals of different ranks use the same
space differently or have access to more or less space depending
on hierarchical seniority. To facilitate surveillance of the appropriate use of space, rank is often displayed by the use of badges,
uniforms, or the equipment carried or used such as a typewrit-
er, stethoscope, or briefcase. This symbolically expressed rank-
ing means that the individual can become invisible to one set of
observers of a different rank while being entirely visible to members of the same rank or below. Therefore, nurses can be visible

to colleagues and to the patients allocated to them while being functionally invisible to medical staff and patients who do not require their services at that time. People of different ranks can perceive the same situation differently in a particular space and time according to their individual perspective and orientation.

The postmodern debate on the cultural effects of space on the way we live our lives can be informative in this regard. An examination of the results of a disruption to physical working conditions demonstrates that our knowledge of the space we inhabit is reflected in our power relations with others who share this space. Nurses who are familiar with the uses of space on a busy ward, including the knowledge of the place where each necessary item of equipment is located, are able to wield power over those who have little knowledge. This power is commonly used through practices of withholding or providing incomplete access to knowledge thereby creating dependence on the owner of the knowledge for the ongoing information necessary to engage in effective clinical practice. These normally transparent power relations become opaque and visible through changed circumstances such as occurs when a ward is moved to a new site. Then the advantage gained by knowing how space is organized and where equipment is kept becomes temporarily negated. Nurses compete to gain knowledge concerning the new location of necessary supplies and equipment and of the restructured uses attributed to particular spaces in the new ward. Resistance to the loss of power/knowledge over space can take the form of disruptive practices such as the arbitary relocation of objects to nondesignated areas or the redesignation of areas of space for different purposes.

Temporality coexists with space to discipline bodies. Work times, such as hospital shifts, are structured into units of time that are allocated particular functions that fit in a formally organized, or informally adhered to, timetables, which include allocated tasks and allocated breaks for meals, use of toilet facilities, etc. Foucault (1975) contends that timetables, whether rigidly imposed or tacitly agreed upon, penetrate the rhythms of the body disciplining and controlling them. Time and space continue to ensure economy of movement in which the whole body is called into play to support the action of one part so that no time is wasted. Bedmaking time is greatly reduced when two nurses cooperate but only if the body of each nurse has been trained to perform the steps in the ritual in sequence and in harmony with each other. Their whole bodies must move in particular predetermined ways, keeping in time, to support the work of the hands.

Disciplining the body requires that the actions manipulate objects in meticulous order in predetermined ways. Time must be used in order not to be "wasted." Therefore, disciplinary procedures provide a constant use of time that pragmatically could be "idle time" by the practice of skill development and the breakdown of skills into a number of set tasks that each take an allotted time. Bedmaking is transcribed into a number of definite unchangeable steps. It is not enough to pull off all the bedclothes at once. Each blanket must be taken off individually and folded neatly before being unfolded to be replaced again. In this way the using of time may provide a false economy of time and labor, however, the body will have been molded into a particular preordained response to the task of bedmaking. Brian Fay (1987:148) describes this process as "transmitting elements of a culture to its newest members by penetrating their bodies directly, without, as it were, passing through the medium of their minds." No wonder bedmaking is described as a mindless task!

According to Foucault (1975), coexisting with disciplines that are easily objectified and analyzed in space, time and movement are those that are less obvious but may impinge more on the lives of those involved in them. This occurs when the disciplines are challenged and become deinstitutionalized, transferred, and adapted. As closed surveillance procedures become deinstitutionalized and extended into community areas, data becomes available for research, which impinges on the private lives and civil liberties of ordinary people. This information can be used in a number of ways to normalize conditions that should be subject to moral or ethical debate, and, as Foucault reminds us, it becomes public property to be used in other coercive ways by the state and other institutions of domination.

Foucault's concept of the disciplines of the body challenges the contention of critical theorists such as Habermas that reflection and collaborative rational discourse will lead to transformative action. As Bordo (1989:13) reminds us, the body is a medium of culture, a text of culture, a metaphor for culture, and a "*practical*, direct locus of social control." We are not disembodied sources of rational thought but people who inhabit real bodies, which are constructed and constrained by our history and which are embedded in a specific culture. Fay (1987:146) challenges us to recognize that "oppression leaves its traces not just in people's minds, but in their muscles and skeletons as well." According to McLaren (1988b:61):

> words and symbols are physiognomic and just as much part of our bodies as our flesh...Discourses do not sit on the surface of the flesh or float about in the formless ether of the mind but are enfolded into the very structures of our desire inasmuch as desire itself is formed by the anonymous historical rules of discourse.

In order to engage in emancipatory praxis it is crucial that the relationship between our rational will, our desires, our experience, and our bodies be established and placed under the scrutiny of critical reflection. This process of reflection will demonstrate the heritage of our position in a society that has been constructed upon the assumptions of duality inherent in a mind/body split. As I have argued elsewhere, this heritage leaves us unable to be

> fully rational and disinterested in a collaborative search for absolute and unversalized, fundamental moral and political principles. The values which we hold, both consciously and unconsciously, and the ways which we have thought and acted prior to this time and place are inscribed upon our bodies ...We have learnt to see our bodies as biological cages which hold our inner thinking self. This concept of duality is hard to unlearn. It permeates our thoughts and actions so that we accept societal constructions within nursing. Rather than examining the phenomena of nursing so that the integral interelationship of our minds and bodies are known and accepted, we tend to examine our thought processes and actions independently. Minds and bodies are distinctly different entities but these entities are inexorably merged through nursing practices. (Street 1990:22)

A weakness in Foucault's telling analysis of the body is the fact that it is predicated upon an assumption that the body is a male body. The female body as an object of disciplinary practices is assumed to be consisent with the male body. There is an inference that the experience of the male body represents the totality of the concept of the body; so the concept of a gendered body is disregarded. Bordo (1989:13) argues that the bodies of women are subject to greater oppression than the bodies of men through the societal practices of making Foucault's concept of "docile bodies" a reality. She argues that as women reentering the public arena they are spending more time on the management and discipline of their bodies than for a very long time. She contends that:

> Through the pursuit of an ever-changing, homogenizing, elusive ideal of femininity—a pursuit without a terminus, a resting point, requiring that women constantly attend to minute and often whimsical changes in fashion...Through the exacting and normalizing disciplines of diet, make-up, and dress—central organizing principles of time and space in the days of many women—we are rendered less socially oriented and more centripetally focused on self-modification. Through these disciplines, we continue to memorize on our bodies the feel and conviction of lack, insufficiency, of never being good enough. At the fartherest extremes, the practices of femininity may lead us to utter demoralization, debilitation, and death. (p.14)

Dimen (1989:38) argues that this focus on self is constructed and perpetuated through the differential experiences of men and women. The use of male nouns and pronouns as the generic form enables men's experience of themselves to be continuous and consistent with their experience of being human. Women's experience, either consciously or unconsciously, is the experience of being both human and other. She contends:

> Culture makes women both human and nonhuman, and they know it, and they must both swallow and reject what they know in order to go from day to day.

I would suggest that no analysis of nursing practice can afford to ignore gender, and no critical analysis of nursing knowledge and action can afford to ignore the concept of the gendered body. According to Connell (1987:87), the concept of a gendered body occurs not only at a symbolic level but at a material level, a level which owns that "the body is never outside history, and history is never free of bodily presence and effects on the body." This concept of the gendered body as located within history and as a socially construction enables Connell (1987:83) to claim:

> The body-as-used, the body I am, is a social body that has taken meanings rather than conferred them. My male body does not confer masculinity on me; it receives masculinity (or some fragment thereof) as its social definition.

Through overt socialization the gendered body is taught the male and female constructed attitudes and actions deemed gender appropriate. Through the process of latent socialization, they also learn those roles and relationships that their culture deems unsuitable for a member of their gender (Lipman-Blumen 1984).

To develop an emancipatory focus in an analysis of clinical nursing practice, it will be necessary to acknowledge a debt to Habermas's concept of the interrelationship of theory and practice as developed through a praxis formed by systematic committed action, which arises from critical reflection. This reflection uncovers both the meaning of the action and a critique of the processes of formation of the meaning, an ideology critique. Through these processes, Habermas contends that emancipatory knowledge will be discovered as a basis for emancipatory action, which then becomes the basis for further reflection and praxis. A debt is also owed to the insights gained from Foucault's geneological approach to power/knowledge enabling us to disclose the power relations, which shape and limit our sociocultural world. A debt is owed to the work of those theorists who have expounded the concepts of critical pedagogy in order to examine the cultural and political processes and structures, which subjugate and resist power relations while providing a language of hope to describe a shared social vision. A further debt needs to be attributed to the work of feminists who critique the implicit patriarchy in the work of social philosophers whose theories are created from a generic concept that equates *person* with *man*, thereby ignoring the empowering capacities and relationships of values such as nurturance.

8

❦

Planning the Route

If you came this way,
Taking the route you would be likely to take
From the place you would be likely to come from

T. S. Eliot, *Little Gidding*

Explorers do not embark on their journeys without extensive preparations. When all available information about the
terrain through which the explorer will travel has been considered, the important task of planning the most appropriate
route through the terrain is commenced. This journey of exploration into the realm of nursing practice required me to examine some of the elements of a research methodology based on
critical social science as a precursor to the decision on my chosen methodology—critical ethnography.

The Choice of an Emancipatory Methodology

Lather (1985) argues that the development of emancipatory
social theory requires a methodology that is

> open-ended, dialogically reciprocal, grounded in a para-
> doxical respect for human capacity and a profound skepti-
> cism of appearances and "common sense," and a commit-
> ment to the long term, broad based ideological struggle
> necessary to transform structural inequalities. (Lather
> 1985:30)

She contends that critical theory with its emancipatory intent provides a powerful and sustained argument of advocacy for the oppressed as a response to the privilege accrued through the perpetuation of the myth of neutral and objective knowledge production and legitimation. This study is located in what Lather (1986) describes as a critical/praxis-oriented research paradigm. This research program is the result of a paradigmatic shift that has moved beyond positivistic research, with its basis in unproblematized claims of scientific neutrality, and beyond naturalistic, interpretive research, which accepts the notion of a socially constructed and negotiated reality but ignores the problems of false consciousness and the mystification produced by ideology. The move to research located within a critical paradigm recognizes the political nature of any knowledge production and legitimating process and argues for a deliberate and acknowledged political agenda aimed at developing emancipatory knowledge. An emancipatory research program recognizes the contradictions inherent in social understandings and in the social order and specifically seeks to locate counterhegemonic practices at work (Giroux 1983). Lather argues that praxis-oriented researchers need to confront issues of empirical accountability if they are not to be accused of the rampant subjectivity of more phenomenological and overtly political research that finds what it is predisposed to look for.

McRobbie (1982) argues that if research is going to change the way that people know and understand things and to challenge the structures that determine their oppressive conditions, then it has to be convincing. She argues against feminists who, in rejecting male-dominated research practice, favor feminine qualities like "intuition, imagination and 'feel'" in the place of "rigour, scholarliness, precision and lucidity" (McRobbie 1982:54). However, McRobbie is not arguing that rigorous and scholarly research is represented by purportedly value-free, quantitative research. Rather, her concern is that feminists and others interested in emancipatory research need to focus on basic issues such as "who we are writing for and why" (McRobbie 1982:54).

This concern for research methods, which are relevant to the research participants as well as to the research audience, is a key area of discussion for those concerned with empowering research. This focus on empowerment affects the nature of the relationship between the researcher and the researched. Lather (1984a) stresses the importance of identifying and rejecting the patronizing stance taken by researchers who do not expect that the respondents will be able to understand the inferences made from the data that they have collaborated in producing. She suggests that critical social researchers who take this stance are no different from the "rape model" of researchers characteristic of mainstream research where career advancement in the social sciences are built on alienating and exploitative methods. McRobbie *(1982)* accuses these researchers of

> prioritizing 'intellectual work'—the eventual book, or even the apriori theory and its fit with the material—over the politics of the situation they leave behind. (1982:51)

The intent of any research based on a critical social science would consciously aim to enable participants to understand and change their situations (Lather 1985). According to Bodemann (1978), the primary focus of any ethically appropriate field methodology can only be the end of the misery which it observes. Therefore, a critical social science methodology accepts the necessity for self-determination by the subjects of the research. Bodemann (1978) quotes Sol Tax, who argues that

> to impose our choices on the assumption that "we know better than they what is good for them" not only restricts their freedom, but it is likely to turn out to be empirically wrong. The point is that what is best for them involves what they want to be. (Bodemann 1978:378)

Lather (1985) reminds us that explicitly value-based research is neither more or less ideological than either positivist or interpretive research, but it does make its interests explicit rather than leave them implicit. This acceptance of subjectivity in research opens the way for the researcher to openly reflect, not only on the research data but on the research methodology and on the values and understandings that the researcher brings to the research.

No research is carried out in a vacuum, and so the questions that we ask and the way in which they are framed is influenced by the historical moment we inhabit (McRobbie 1982). It is important to recognize that the actual conventions of the research process itself are socially constructed in much the same way as the sociocultural world in which the research is located. This means that research activities such as writing, interviewing, case studies, and theory building are tasks that need to be demystified and open to discussion and contestation. Lather (1985:32) argues that when the issue is recognized as the problem of the "neutrality of data rather than researcher, unabashedly ideological research no longer need apologize for its open commitment to using research to critique and change the status quo."

This aspect is explored by McRobbie (1982) who argues that attention should be given to the ideological nature and partiality of any account. She suggests that emancipatory researchers often use their subjects as arbitrators by letting them speak out for themselves. She questions the assumption that this kind of reporting produces something "pure" or "definitive" because recorded speech goes through a number of transformations before it is included in a research report. Even when not juxtaposed with the researcher's comments and analyses, recorded speech is separated from its social and historical context, is deliberately chosen by the researchers as against other possible excerpts, and as such is ideologically loaded (Polkinghorne 1983).

McRobbie (1982), in her discussion on research methodologies for feminist research, looks at the dilemma that the oral tradition of women poses for researchers. She argues that "we all talk, all of the time," but few people "dare distil from all our discussions and arguments, the theories and analyses presented in print" (1982:50). She contends that women are encultured into an oral tradition; therefore, emancipatory research must identify and support the need for a political (and obviously, personal) struggle to break free from the privatized confines of talk to an engagement in the public sphere through written records and research.

This is particularly relevant to research into nursing because traditionally nursing has been written about by a small group of nurse scholars. In Victoria the recent nurse's strike has changed the public and private face of nursing. It has begun a process that has provided rank-and-file nurses with the opportunity (and the luxury of time that the enforced rest from work combined with constant attendance at stop work meetings has provided) to talk about nursing. This dis-

covery of talk as consciousness-raising has developed a solidarity and a way of defining relationships between nurses that
has enabled many nurses to make the transition from the private to the public sphere and to engage in overt political struggle. Davis (1986, *The Age*, p.10) describes the all-encompass-
ing effect on the whole range of nurses when he writes:

> It is clear that at a personal level, the strike has radical-
> ized the thousands of mainly middle-class women who
> have been involved.

This public engagement in the debate and political action
needs to flow over into recording and research processes,
which embrace all nurses, so that the "elite" scholars are no
longer left with this task. The intent of research into nursing
based on a critical social science would consciously aim to
enable the participants (nurses) to critique the oppressive elements in their situations as a basis for change. This concept of
collaborative and emancipatory research begins with the problems of the participants and proceeds through a process of
action and reflection to an understanding of, and ability to
change, the social situation that oppresses them; it is in this
process that people change themselves and their understandings of themselves.

Tandon (1981) argues that this research process gives
ordinary people power to redefine the purpose of knowledge
and to influence the generation, utilization and dissemination
of knowledge as the basis upon which they can act to counter
oppression. Within the research process ideas evolve from the
insights of practice, become systematized into theory and tested in practice as the basis for further theory development and
ongoing radical action. This cyclical, evolutionary process is
central to empowering research methodologies.

The selection of an appropriate methodology for critical
praxis-oriented research is governed by a number of factors.
These include the social and political constraints of the chosen
field setting, the time and resources available, the feasibility of
the research design, the purpose of the study, and the relationship of the researcher to the researched whether peer or
"outsider." After careful consideration of the options and the
factors mentioned, I chose to use critical ethnography for this
proposed study on nursing.

Ethnography as a Basis for Critical Ethnography

This section introduces and examines the rationale, structure, and methods of an ethnography as the basis for a later exposition of critical ethnography. Ethnography is a research method of the interpretive sciences and as such cannot be the basis of openly ideological critical social science. However, in the same way that an understanding of interpretive methods is necessary for the paradigmatic shift to the critical paradigm, ethnography forms the basis upon which critical ethnography is posited.

According to Wilson (1977), the rationale for the use of ethnographic techniques is based on two sets of hypotheses about human behavior. The naturalistic-ecological hypothesis is concerned with a commitment to the idea that the study of human behavior should be subject to the influences of the natural setting and not the specialized influences resulting from the contrived research setting. The qualitative-phenomenological hypothesis emphasizes the necessity for the researcher to search for the meanings that participants place on their behavior. In order to be consistent with these hypotheses, it is necessary for the researcher to engage in observation in the field and to participate with the research participants in a process of clarification of the meanings of observed behaviors. Wilson argues that ethnography is based on the assumption that what people say and the way they behave is shaped, consciously and unconsciously, by their social situation. Stenhouse (1985) supports this view by arguing that the "outsider" is able to challenge the apparent understandings of the participants by disclosing and providing explanations that highlight the causal and structural patterns that they experience.

Ethnography is practiced across a number of academic disciplines, and consequently there is considerable diversity in elucidating its distinctive features. Spradley (1979) regards ethnography as the vehicle for a detailed description and analysis of cultural knowledge. A different emphasis narrows the focus to the investigation of patterns of social interaction within a cultural field (Grumperz 1981). Another perspective argues for ethnography as encompassing a holistic analysis of cultures or social orders (Lutz 1981).

For the purposes of this study ethnography is characterized as an in-depth, long-term case study carried out by a researcher who is an outsider to the field setting and who engages in an intensive examination of a specific situation, which enables the researcher to identify basic phenomena as a basis for theory development (Kenny 1984). The ethnographer participates in the lives of the research participants for an extended length of time observing, recording, questioning, and collecting data for analysis.

The ethnographer does not approach the field with a specific hypotheses to be tested. Glaser and Strauss (1967) have argued for an open attitude to the field in which the ethnographer engages in systematic data collection as a basis for the identification of theories for validity testing in the field. Others have argued for a good training in theory, and an acquaintance with the issues of the field, as the basis for the development of valuable theory from the phenomena recorded in the field (Malinowski 1922; Hammersley 1983).

The literature surrounding the methodology of ethnography engages in arguments designed to define the role of the participant-observer (e.g., Gans 1967; Gold 1958). Some writers are concerned with the competing claims of the researcher as observer and participant. This discussion revolves around contentions concerned with the extent to which the researcher is acting a role as an observer as opposed to a competing role as a participant, and the interrelationship between the two roles. The issue at stake here is a concern to represent and understand the values and actions of the research participants while retaining the status of evaluator. This is consistent with interpretive research, which endeavors to uncover the meanings of the situation in such a way that the participants can identify and understand the issues. The rationale behind this approach enables the researcher's task to end with the enlightenment of the participants concerning their present situation and the way in which history and tradition have caused and shaped it. The ethnographer recognizes the place of values in the researcher role and uses these to increase understanding but also participates in a distancing process in the theory-building and reporting stage.

The conduct of an ethnography differs from researcher to researcher and from discipline to discipline. There are a number of generic concepts that can be expected to be examined within an ethnographic study. The need to select an appropriate field site and negotiate access to it is a process that requires the location of sponsors, to provide introductions, and gatekeepers, who have the main control over key resources and access to people and places within the field site. Many ethnographers begin with a pilot or sampling phase as the basis for more informed choices of appropriate informers as research participants. This process not only enables the researcher to engage participants who will be the most useful to the research in terms of strategic experience and information but also to check that these people are indeed representative of the group and not atypical.

Although the main method of data collection for an ethnographer will be the compilation of descriptive field notes through the process of participant observation, these notes will be supported by other methods such as in-depth interviews and documentation from records and reports to achieve triangulation of the data. In this way the researcher can check the inferences from one set of data against the inferences developed from another (Smith 1983; Wilson 1977). An important source of data validation will come from the research participants themselves. According to Hammersley (1983), ethnographic data analysis begins with a thorough reading of the data to gain enough familiarity to use the data to think with. He suggests that this process uncovers patterns and relationships between the data and common-sense knowledge, official reports, and previous theory. It also highlights discrepancies, contradictions, and inconsistencies between espoused views and action. This thinking develops analytic categories as the basis for theoretical frameworks. The data can then be examined in detail for the identification of typologies, which can provide the link between the data and the emerging concepts as a basis for theory development.

The writing of ethnographies requires decisions about style and content, chronology and analytical frameworks. Ethnographers need to include detailed cultural descriptions and narratives to substantiate the analysis and theory building. Style decisions reflect commitments to different emphases. Ethnographic portrayals may appear as a form of storytelling (Walker 1982; Hymes 1978), whereas another emphasis may organize the work in a number of themes (Hamilton 1977; Whyte 1981), another narrows and expands the focus through analytical stages (Lacey 1970), and another separates the narration from analysis (Willis 1977).

Critical Ethnography: Politics, Reciprocity, and Reflection

Critical ethnography is a recent development in research methodologies and, as such, has been documented rarely and incompletely. Even Willis's (1977) classic critical ethnography—*Learning to Labor*—provides limited elucidation of his methodological rationale and lacks a theoretical description of a critical ethnography. This lack of documentation limits my capacity to provide a comprehensive overview of a critical ethnography and provides me with a challenge to participate in the further development of this research methodology.

A critical ethnography develops from a commitment to an emancipatory critical social science designed to empower the research participants and to engage in a process of collectively developed emancipatory theory building (Lather 1984a). This approach accepts the role of values in research and openly explicates its own values, which focus on a commitment to uncover the causal mechanisms of oppression, and through collaborative rational dialogue and reflection, work to bring about change. The critical ethnographer is not able to hide behind the facade of the research role, but takes an advocacy role that enables the participants to work toward their own liberation from oppressive structures.

A crucial element of a critical ethnography is the collaborative process. In an ethnography the onus is on the researcher to identify and describe the phenomena and to develop the theory from the insight and understandings of the participants, whereas in a critical ethnography the research participants share in this task and, in the process, have their actions and understandings challenged. An ethnographer endeavors to use the data to develop the perspective needed to theorize about the issues in the setting, whereas a critical ethnographer has a paradigmatic commitment to openly value-based, advocacy research and, as such, a commitment to collaboration with research participants in problem posing and theory development. Therefore, the difference between an ethnography and a critical ethnography can be highlighted by an examination of the role of the critical ethnographer. Rather than describing this role as a variation on the participant/ observer label, I have found it convenient to think of the role as a militant observer. In using the term *militant*, I am seeking to explain the openly ideological nature of the role that leads to and supports active intervention in the field setting. Bodemann (1978:409) describes this as "interventive observation" and argues that most sociologists "seem unaware or blind to the fact that the interaction of the researcher with the field is a political issue." He argues that ethnographic work "has become of paramount importance given the sophisticated manipulation of our lives today" because an extended critique can guide us to "politically and methodologically adequate approaches to field work" (1978:410).

Using Marx's account of his early British researchers in the Enquete Ouvriere, Bodemann (1978:410) develops guidelines to describe the role of the researcher involved in "intervention observation" as:

1. He(/She) participates fully, freely and self-critically in the setting.

2. He(/She) observes and renders a description of the facts and "on-goings" of the setting, but in the context of his(/her) biographical position...

3. Given his commitment and the evidence, received and theoretically grounded, he(/she) can actively intervene: first by presenting options to a community which has been deprived of options, divided and paralysed,...second, by returning his(/her) findings (descriptive and theoretical) to the community, by sharing it with others who partake in a comparable predicament and with all those who identify with this predicament and who are willing to change it.

Although these guidelines were developed for a researcher who would participate fully by sharing the activities in the field setting, as occurs in participatory research, they are also helpful in providing insights into the role of the critical ethnographer. Jennings (1986:9) argues that critical ethnographic case studies differ from ethnography by allowing both the researcher and the research participants to become active in and conscious of the process of change through ideology critique and self-reflection. She claims that through this process participants within the case studies become empowered to make their own decisions.

I believe that a critical ethnography is an appropriate methodology for research into nursing. This process enables the researcher to collaborate with nurses in their own enlightenment by identifying the key issues involved in their emancipation from the power/knowledge relations that shape, mold and limit their rational pursuit of justice in nursing. The commitment to the development of a case study over the period of time enables the researcher to be active in the cyclical process of observation, collaborative data analysis, reflection, and theory making.

According to Boud (1985), the reflection process begins with the goal to reconstruct experience as a basis for understanding the attitudes and emotions that shape our knowledge of the world and as a basis for incorporating new ideas and information. He argues that reflection is not merely daydreaming or idle speculation but is an activity that is both purposeful and goal-directed. Kemmis (1985:140) argues that reflection is not "a purely 'internal,' psychological process: it is action-oriented and historically embedded." He suggests that this is a dialectic process in which reflection looks both inward at the person and outward to the situation. Both the personal and situational aspects of reflection have been been shaped by historical processes. According to Kemmis, we do not reflect in a vacuum but in response to a given situation. The reflection process is a social process because the ideas and understandings that we generate from our reflection are socially constructed and the actions that flow from these understandings are similarly shaped and constrained by society.

The reflection process then reconstructs actions and experiences, which are recorded for analysis. This analytical process not only uncovers the personal and nursing issues and meanings at work in the situation but uncovers the historical and social factors that have shaped both the nurse and the clinical setting. This analysis forms the basis of a problem-setting exercise where problems are posed to enable the nurse to question the tacit ways of knowing and practicing nursing. This confrontation of experiences, and of the meanings and assumptions that surround them, can form a foundation upon which to make choices about future actions, based on chosen value stances and new ways of thinking about, and understanding, nursing practice.

In his work on professional education Schön (1983) found that professionals often engage in what he describes as "reflection-in-action" or "a reflective conversation with the situation."

They may structure the reflection so that others, such as students or fellow workers, participate and "think along" with them, and the reflection becomes a collaborative process. However, according to Schön, professionals seldom reflect upon their reflection-in-action so "this crucially important dimension...tends to remain private and inaccessible to others" (1983:243).

As this study challenges some of the the taken-for-granted assumptions in nursing culture through the process of critical reflection, it is appropriate that this same process of critical reflection should be used to critically examine the research process itself. This would provide a critical engagement with the paradigm and methodology of the study. A critical reflection can uncover the historical and traditional constraints that shaped the research process and identify the social and political interests that have been served by the research. Openly ideological critical social science explicates its emancipatory values and interests, and the role that these values played in guiding the research would need critical reflection.

9

❦

Exploring the Uncharted Country

Any journey into an unknown region needs to take account of the possibilities and potentialities of the country. A foray into the uncharted country of clinical nursing practice requires planning. However, even the best laid plans can come astray, and for this reason the choice of a research site and the strategies involved in setting up the research require some attention.

The Research Site: Exploratory Phase

The research project began with an exploratory stage during which time a number of options were canvassed and considered as to their suitability as sites for the conduct of the research. The options under consideration were an acute general hospital, a nonacute private hospital, a geriatric nursing home, a group of community health nurses based in community health centers, and a similar group of maternal and child health nurses. Preliminary discussions with, and observation of, nurses engaged in these settings provided the opportunity to collect data on nursing practice in these varied settings and to use that data to identify common issues of relevance to most nurses as distinct from those issues that are context and role specific to specialist nurses in specific settings.

During this exploratory stage it became apparent that nurses engaged in the nonacute nursing home and community-based settings had more autonomy in nursing actions and directions. This increased autonomy had been deliberately sought out by the nurses working in these settings and was often described in terms of their survival as nurses.

> I just would not go back to working in an acute hospital, I wouldn't survive. I was so glad to escape from hospitals and get into community nursing. At least here you can organize your own work and make your own decisions about the best things for your client. (RN, Community Health)

The drift of experienced clinical nurses from the acute hospital settings to the nonacute and specialist areas is reflected in the kinds of nursing research that emanates from acute and nonacute settings. Research into nursing in acute settings tends to be medically oriented and empirically designed, whereas research in nonacute settings appear to have provided the very limited amount of qualitative research into nursing practice. This tendency has developed because in acute settings research has to be negotiated with a number of gatekeepers and be conducted within the constraints and expectations of a medically oriented hierarchical setting. Many of the gatekeepers of acute research settings are doctors or administrators whose understanding of research is grounded in the positivist paradigm and its methods. They generally support empirical nursing research because it is consistent with their views of research practice and because it generally addresses questions of interest to medicine and administration as well as to nursing.

By contrast the nurses in nonacute and community settings tend to be more experienced clinical practitioners interested in the kind of questions about nursing practice that require qualitative methods to provide satisfactory answers. Qualitative research is more easily conducted in settings where the nurse has a large measure of control over the gatekeeping process and has access to structured settings such as a long-term chronic ward or a number of regular appointments with a client or client group.

I decided to work with nurses in both an acute setting, and a nonacute setting but my experience of the difficulties of observing nurses in the acute setting led me to recognize that I would need to make a choice. Therefore, I chose to conduct my research in an acute general hospital because this is where the majority of nurses are employed and yet this area has been generally neglected by qualitative researchers. Although an acute hospital is a difficult setting in which to conduct research, particularly for a nurse employee who is relatively powerless within the system, or for an outsider such as myself, it is also the most appropriate site for an examination of the way in which clinical nurses make sense of their practice within power/knowledge relationships.

Choice of a Research Site

I decided to approach a large general teaching hospital, which provided the clinical medical school for an established university with an accompanying research unit. This hospital provided hospital-based education for nurses at a basic and postbasic level and provided clinical placements for college educated nurses. The hospital administration had recently employed a nurse-researcher to coordinate those research projects in the hospital that used nurses or whose subject matter related to nursing. The director of nursing was known to be interested in educational research.

Negotiated Access: Gatekeepers and Sponsors

The process of obtaining access to the research setting necessitated engaging in formal and informal procedures. As Hammersley (1983) suggests, this process is more difficult in those formal settings where boundaries are clearly marked and are policed by gatekeepers. He reminds us that in formal bureaucratic organizations there is often a blurring between gatekeepers and sponsors and that it is often not obvious whose permission needs to be obtained or whose support needs to be solicited. It is also difficult for an outsider to understand the unwritten procedures, which support the formalized written procedures, and to identify informal sources of power, which may not appear to have a corresponding formalized authority within the hierarchy. Successful entry into the public hospital necessitated the identification of sponsors who would act as informants for me concerning formal and informal processes of access and the identification of gatekeepers who had the authority to legitimate my entry and provide support.

My first contact was with a nursing supervisor who, as a

member of the middle management of the hospital, was able to act as an informant concerning formal and informal processes. This woman was known to me and was very interested in my research topic and in qualitative nursing research. She then acted as a sponsor by speaking on my behalf to the nurse-researcher, employed by the hospital, to find out the correct official procedure. The nurse-researcher contacted me and explained that I should begin the process by writing a formal letter of introduction to the director of nursing requesting an interview to discuss my proposed research. I wrote a letter of introduction and included copies of my references from previous research and work in similar field settings; I had been told that this would be advantageous because I was not a nurse.

The formal letter was then passed from the director of nursing to the nurse-researcher for assessment and advice prior to the requested interview. In this way the nurse-researcher was incorporated into the gatekeeping role of the director. In the role of gatekeeper the nurse-researcher arranged a time to discuss my research. She was unfamiliar with qualitative research and was unsure of the consequences for the hospital and staff in my request to follow individual nurses around twice a week over a nine-month period. She explained that the hospital staff were used to research based on physical measurement or one-off questionnaires and that she could not predict the reaction to my request for access by either the director of nursing or the hospital research committee, which included medical and administrative staff. I provided her with a short resume of my proposal and the ethical procedures that would govern the conduct of the research. Discussions continued firstly with the nurse-researcher and then between her and the nursing supervisor who was acting as my sponsor. The nurse-researcher was particularly interested in how I would be able to measure and standardize the data. She expressed the view that nurses were choosing to do qualitative research because they perceived it as being easier. I assured her that good qualitative research was not easier, a point with which she would now concur. These discussions culminated in the organization of a meeting with the director of nursing.

This meeting was brief and highly successful for me as the director of nursing approved of my research proposal and offered any support that I would need including access to hospital reports and membership of the medical library. This support later enabled me to be allowed access to a parking space in the free medical car park in the hospital grounds. The director of nursing was particularly interested in my topic, which had become more topical as a result of the 1986 RANF strike and the subsequent inquiry into the issues of clinical nursing practice. At that point in the history of nursing in Victoria, the nursing shortage was acute, and nurses were developing a much higher political and public profile. Any inquiry that might provide new knowledge about nursing practice while not costing the hospital was potentially useful. It was also apparent that the director of nursing had more knowledge of, and experience with, qualitative research than her staff.

This acceptance by the director of nursing turned the previously cautious gatekeeping nurse-researcher into a sponsor who facilitated the next access processes. She provided advice on the format and content of my proposal to the next set of gatekeepers, the hospital research committee, and supported my proposal in the discussions at that meeting which enabled me to gain permission to conduct my research at the hospital. She furnished me with organizational support such as the procurement of access to the previously mentioned car space, some shared office space, and access to the photocopier. She also provided me with a great deal of general information about the hospital through informal discussions, a guided tour, and copies of nursing reports, procedures manual and submissions to government inquiries.

The nurse-researcher was concerned that the approach to nurses was handled through her and undertook to obtain two nurses for me to work with initially. She spoke with each nurse individually and then organized a meeting for me to meet with the nurses and herself in her office. This meeting enabled me to explain my research objectives and to present each of the nurses with the principles of procedures document and to explain it thoroughly to them. One of these nurses was the RANF union key representative, who not only had access to all the hospital nursing staff and the key issues of contention but had also participated in other nursing research and was very interested in research. The other nurse was a very experienced charge nurse, who had worked in the hospital for over a decade at a senior level and who had spent some months on secondment to the hospital school of nursing before returning to work in charge on the wards. These two nurses both agreed to be involved in the research project and also acted as sponsors in my introduction to other staff and wards.

The support of all these sponsors proved invaluable as they were senior enough to have access to the informal and formal processes of entry to the site but were also actively involved in nursing practice and/or research and so were able to introduce me to the informal networks of clinical nurses in the hospital.

Selection of Research Participants: Mutual Engagement

The hospital nurse-researcher and I agreed to begin the research with a pilot phase based around the two selected nurses and the wards in which they were involved. This would provide some boundaries for me as I began to orient myself to the nursing culture and to collect detailed observations of nursing practices. This decision also facilitated a process enabling the nurse-researcher to monitor my work as it was an entirely new kind of research activity for the hospital.

After the pilot phase was completed, I had intended to include nurses from other wards in the research in order to provide as much variety in nursing actions. However, during the pilot phase it soon became clear that the rosters, shift arrangements, education days, and holidays of these nurses coupled with my own limitations of university commitments and personal life meant that it would be very difficult to develop in-depth profiles on a number of wards. I also realized that this approach would not enable me to differentiate the personal nursing styles and idiosyncratic responses to particular nursing issues as I would not have comparisons and multiple interpretations of the same action and situation. I decided that it would be beneficial to include other nurses from the same wards in the pilot phase and then make more informed choices of five nurses for the study itself. This meant that instead of following a number of nurses from a variety of wards I concentrated on nurses from a busy medical ward and the intensive care ward. In my choices of nurses I was guided by the charge nurses of both wards, both of whom offered to participate in the research. I asked for nurses from varied backgrounds and experience, which meant that the work experience of the final group ranged from a new graduate to a nurse with over twenty years of ongoing nursing experience, as well as including nurses who had been educated in different hospitals and college courses with different styles and philosophies of nurse education.

The nurses used in this pilot phase were given copies of the information concerning the principles of procedure and agreed to allow me to observe them and discuss the material with them. They felt that they would then be in a better position to decide if they were prepared to participate in the larger study. The wider range of nurses participating in the pilot phase enabled me to make decisions about the kind of nurses I would work with in the study. I found that my initial decision to work with nurses ranging from a new graduate to a senior charge nurse would not provide me with as much information on the power/knowledge issues in nursing practice as a group of experienced nurses. During the pilot phase it became apparent that neophyte nurses and even those with some experience, tended to focus on the mastery of skills, routines, and complexities in order to become a proficient nurse able to act appropriately within the nursing culture. This focus meant that they not only found it difficult to isolate and examine nursing issues that arose from their nursing actions but found it a confusing and generally unsatisfactory process. By contrast I found that the experienced nurses were able to readily identify key issues and able to work creatively with me in the process of locating the power/knowledge relations at work within their adherence to certain habits, myths, and routinized actions in their practice. In an attempt to develop a study that had enough boundaries and limitations to procure sufficient in-depth data for analysis and theory development, I chose to use five experienced nurses as case study research participants in this critical ethnographic study.

The recruitment process of the five nurses provided me with insights into the role of the charge nurses and the nurse-researcher. The charge nurses were accustomed to a role of being in authority in relation to their nurses and took the initiative to convene meetings to enable me to talk with the appropriate staff members that I was intending to recruit without further reference to me or the nursing researcher. This was easy and sensible, but I had agreed that the nurse-researcher was to set up the contacts and to be present at the initial meetings. To resolve this I ended up having informal discussions with staff at the meetings convened by the charge nurses but then explained that this was an official research project and that my own self-imposed rules of procedure required that they be recruited officially, which meant another meeting in the presence of the nurse-researcher in which they would receive copies of the principles of procedure and at which time all of the implications and expectations of the research would be fully explained. I then arranged these meetings with the charge nurse and nurse-researcher. The charge nurses were obviously mystified as to why I was adopting such a formal process and as to why the nurse-researcher needed to be present. I also found the process frustrating because it entailed a formality that was in opposition to the informal relations that I had already developed with these staff but it highlighted for me the bounds and ethics of the research.

The pilot phase also enabled the nurses who were to participate in the case studies time to get to know me and my methods and to decide if they wanted to work with me and take responsibility in engaging in mutual reciprocity within the research. Some nurses soon recognized that they did not want to take the time out of working hours or the responsibility of negotiating interpretations of the data with me. Others, however, became very interested and in making my choice I looked for experienced clinical nurses who were able to analyze nursing issues and had already begun to think about their clinical practices in the light of these issues. As this recruitment process was occurring not long after the RANF strike, each of the women chosen was able to talk about the radicalizing effect on themselves as nurses and their heightened consciousness of nursing issues. However, each nurse in the study had been subject to very different professional experiences and influences and had different interests in nursing practice.

During the pilot phase I observed and took notes about nursing actions engaged in by a variety of nurses from a medical ward and an intensive care ward in the hospital. As some of the new graduates were moved temporarily to other wards, I was able to see them in action in different contexts. This material was structured so that it was not identifiable. Comments on the data by the participating nurses tended to be focused on elaboration, correction, and interpretation of the data rather than any in-depth analysis.

The beginning of the ethnographic case studies marked the end of these generalized observations and the start of a process of limiting my written observations of action to nurses in the wards to those who were active participants in the research, and with whom I was committed to joint ownership of the data that related to them. Initially this boundary seemed to be limiting when I was in a situation to observe a number of nurses who had become interested in my research and were offering me the opportunity to make observations of them also. After thinking through the implications of having free access to all the nurses on a ward I decided that the value of this research lay in the depth of meaning made jointly by myself and the research participants. As my research focus was issues-based, I decided that observation of the participants in their interactions with other nurses, staff and patients over a long period of time would enable me to uncover the nursing issues and develop the relationships within which to discuss them. The fact that four nurses in the case studies were expecting to move to another hospital or to be moved to another ward about halfway through the research process would enable us to evaluate our data and understandings of the issues that we had raised in the work on the previous ward. However, the opportunity to spend at least six months on two very different wards meant that I was able to be immersed in the specific nursing culture of those wards before taking a more general view in relation to other wards in this hospital and in other hospitals.

Data Collection: Negotiated Strategies

The deliberate interactive design of this critical ethnography enabled the nurses to negotiate the data collection strategies. This interactive, reflexive negotiation changed the research design from one based on the written word to one that took equal account of the oral basis to nursing culture. Where I had intended that the nurses would keep responding to my written work with their own written responses, I found that they were reluctant to write much more than explanations, corrections, and comments. However, they were very ready to talk about what I had found and what they had read in the data, so I began to record and tape conversations at length for later transcription and analysis.

The data collection strategies can be described in a number of distinct but overlapping phases.

Exploratory Phase. During this phase I began to observe

and discuss nursing practices with a number of nurses from different settings. These notes and observations confirmed for me my desire to engage in a critical ethnography of nursing practices and informed my subsequent decision to work in an acute general hospital. During the process of negotiating access to the hospital, I was able to read a history of the hospital, a number of submissions prepared by the hospital for government inquiries, the procedures manual, and a number of reports relating to nursing in the hospital.

Pilot Phase. During this phase I began observation of two nurses who had leadership roles in two different wards—a medical ward and the intensive care ward. The emphasis of the observation was to develop a general overview of the wards and discover the protocols, routines, and rituals which existed there. The invitation to include observations of other nurses was extended and organized on a short-term basis. This provided a more comprehensive overview of the specificities of the nursing role and the cultural norms in operation as a basis for later identification of the place of role boundaries in nursing resistance.

Nurses are skilled at the use of their senses, and at this time I was encouraged to use my senses to collect information for later note taking rather than attempting to take extensive notes. The process enabled me to immerse myself in the culture of a shift and to ask constant questions. During this time I documented many of the routines and rites, which were later to become almost invisible to me through familiarity. This documentation forms the basis of the practices that were later analyzed to uncover power/knowledge relations at work. My interest in those things that were taken for granted by the nurses amazed them. They had expected me to begin with issues like medical ethics and were surprised that I was questioning basic things like uniforms, rosters, tea breaks, and bedmaking routines. In order to demonstrate the way in which I would work with the seemingly trivial to uncover power/knowledge relations, I wrote a provocative paper on uniforms for distribution to the nurses in the pilot group. This paper formed the basis for explanations on the value of analyzing the habitual, taken-for-granted nursing actions and practices as a way of uncovering larger issues of ethics, medical domination, knowledge control, and the hegemony of male-created science in the development of nursing practice.

Phase 1. The observations taken during this stage were similar to those in the pilot phase, but they were focused narrowly on to the specific nurses chosen for the case study. This process was more difficult than the pilot phase because I would only follow one nurse at a time even if other nurses in the research were also working that shift. This meant that I had to deal with two new factors—mobility and space. This helped me to understand the complexities involved in working in a highly mobile manner in small spaces, which had functioned differently for different staff. If I had placed myself strategically in a corner to observe what I could from that perspective, as is often done in studies of nurses, I would have missed the mobility/space factors. The nurses themselves were unaware of the significance of mobility and space as they were used to structuring their work to take account of them.

The nurses were generally very mobile, particularly on the ward, so I spent a great deal of time following them from one place to another. Sometimes the nurses would tell me where they were going, but once accustomed to my presence, and concentrating on their patients, they would often just disappear in a particular direction with me hurrying after them, and often meeting them on their return with something from a store. It took some time before I could judge if the trip was to be short, enabling me to wait with the patient, or whether by not following I was to lose contact with the nurse for a while. Even when the nurse explained that she was only going to the linen cupboard and that I could chat to the patient until she came back, I soon discovered that she could be delayed and not return for some time. I decided to try to follow along during this phase so that I could see the way in which the nurses organized their time around the needs of the patient, the needs of administration, the paramedics, and the doctors and how they dealt with the constant interruptions to their tasks. Notes were scribbled at odd times and in odd places that were dictated by the need to observe on the run.

I discovered that hospital staff generally conduct their patient care within very limited spaces, which were often shared with others who used them for a different function. These spaces had different symbolic meanings for different staff, patients, and visitors in the same way as the space behind the counter in a shop is symbolically "out of bounds" for customers but not for shop assistants. During this phase I became aware of places that were considered useful to stand and observe and other places that meant that I would be in the way. Often observation places that worked well for the nurse would be found to be intrusive to the work of the medical or paramedical staff. In an intensive care unit space is not only controlled by function but by the complexity of the technological interventions and by invisible barriers, which represent zones of sterility and require different hygiene procedures. This meant that my observations were complicated by the need to learn correct hygienic procedures for specific kinds of contact or proximity to particular kinds of patients. I had to learn when to wash my hands and what kind of protective clothing—gown, plastic apron, or face mask—was appropriate to collect data in that setting and be ready to discard them for another set of procedures when the nurse moved on to another space zone.

The observations made during this stage were often verbatim reports of action and conversations between the nurse and others and the nurse and myself.

A cag's (coronary artery graft) patient needs to have the chest drainage tubes removed. The two tubes are to be removed from the lungs. Ann explains to the patient exactly what she is going to do:

Ann: What I am going to do now is to take out these two drainage tubes out of your lungs, it may hurt a bit but you will feel a lot better after...at least that's what most patients tell me. Now are you in pain?...just a little...OK I am giving you morphine through your drip so I will just give you a little more to help you when I remove the tubes.

Ann adjusted the morphine level and explained to me that the patient had a big chest drain with a tube in the thoracic cavity and a second in the heart sac. The tubes are usually left in for twenty-four hours as had been the case for this patient. Ann then checked on the pain level of the patient. As he was comfortable with the increased morphine in the drip she removed the outer dressings and painted the area with antiseptic.

Ann: Is it sore? You are pretty tough aren't you.

Ann then took off the dressings covering the drainage

tubes and explained the next step to the patient.

Ann: When I tell you that I am ready I want you to take a big breath in...you will feel a bit of a tug but hold on to your breath or you will get air into your lungs where it shouldn't be. OK?

Ann then asks another nurse to scrub and help her. This nurse is experienced with this task and so Ann just says:

Can you help me for a minute? I am going to remove (patient)'s tubes. Can you do the strings for me?

Ann to me: Can you cope with blood as this could be gory? Sometimes the blood spurts out everywhere.

Ann to patient: OK are you ready...Now take a big breath and hold.

Ann quickly removes the first tube and the assisting nurse pulls the drawstrings and ties the stitches. Meanwhile Ann watches the patient and tells him when to breathe out. She disposes of the tube and checks on the patient again. Ann holds his arm and asks.

Ann: Does that feel alright? Are you ready for the next one?

The patient nods. Ann and the other nurse repeat the task. The second time the tube leaks a bit and smells awful. While the nurse is tying the stitches Ann checks on the patient telling him that the smell is normal and then cleans up the mess as quickly as possible.

Ann: Does that feel better now?

The patient nods weakly. As Ann cleans up and checks the patient's monitors she tells him:

I will get another x-ray later. It is routine. We check that when the tubes are removed your lung doesn't collapse down a bit. I will take you to the shower later and get you cleaned up.

Ann takes away soiled towels and the now unnecessary equipment from the bay. She puts a fresh sheet on the patient and moves him into a more comfortable position. The patient tells Ann that he really feels a lot better now. She checks that his pillows and sheet are comfortable and decides to give him a rest.

Ann: OK now, I will turn off the lights and let you rest a bit.

Phase 2. This phase merged with the first phase and became an extension to it, but the distinct aspect of this phase is that it marked the time when I began to feed back what I had been observing to the nurses. Although I offered it in note form, I soon realized that the nurses did not have the time or inclination to read all my notes and observations but that they were happy to sit down during a meal break and listen to me reading and describing the content of my notes and to respond orally to them. The focus of this exercise was clarification of the notes and observations in order to provide a basis for later analysis. The procedure would generally follow a pattern in which I read or described what I had observed and received explanations, challenges, other contextual details and inevitably some useful personal illustrations of actions based on the material under consideration. I would record specific illustrations, quotes, and key summaries to add to the data.

Phase 3. This phase was characterized by detailed observations of actions and conversations. By this time I was familiar with the regular actions and routines in the ward, and I was able to concentrate on particular details and ignore others. I collected very specific information on particular shifts using my watch to time nursing actions as demonstrated in my field notes taken while observing Eve a charge nurse in an intensive care unit.

1:55 p.m.   Eve came back from lunch early. She answered the phone and spoke to the wife of the patient in bay 6. She organized a convenient visiting time.

2:00 p.m.   Eve arranged for the family members of the accident victim (including the husband) who had arrived at the hospital from the country to come to the interview room. She gave them a rundown on what an ICU unit was like physically and how it worked. Eve explained that the patient often looked worse because they were hooked up to monitoring equipment and that could be frightening to their relatives and friends. She then explained what had been done to the patient and the fact that she was not conscious but could possibly hear. She encouraged the relatives to go in with her two at a time and told them she would answer all their questions.

2:10 p.m.   The husband and sister went in with Eve and sobbed as she sat and talked with them quietly. Eve continued to stroke the husband's arm and encouraged him to come closer to his wife and to touch her. He was very reluctant and did not stay in the bay long. She answered the sister's questions and brought in other relatives.

2:20 p.m.   When all the relatives had seen the accident victim in pairs, Eve went into the interview room and answered their questions. She then asked the family for details of the woman's usual habits and reactions to aid the nurses in their diagnosis and care plans. She recorded the information on the nursing care plan and showed it to the nurse in that bay and to the nurse acting in-charge.

2:25 p.m.   Eve returned to the bay as the husband and sister had decided to see the woman again. He motioned Eve to come into the bay but as he was Italian and very upset he had difficulty speaking coherently in English. Eve put her arm around him and kept rubbing his back as she encouraged him to come closer to his wife. She stayed with him as he cried, and when he was calmer she sat him on the other side of the patient where her arm was less injured and encouraged the husband to stroke it and speak to his unconscious wife.

Over time it became apparent that much of the data relating to tasks and routines was repetitious so I tended to only document anything that was new, contradictory to previous data or part of a progression of changing behaviors. During this time I also began to challenge the taken-for-grantedness of the comments that the nurses were using to describe their understandings of clinical practice.

Diane: Nurses need an authoritarian figure to look up to. If they don't get that from the nurse in charge then they get it from an administrator or a doctor.

A.S.: Why do you believe that nurses need to look up to a person in authority.

Diane: I think it may be a female thing. We certainly need a role model.

A.S.: What about male nurses, do they need a role model?

Diane: Yes, I guess it can't just be because we are female. We all need role models to learn.

A.S.: I am confused about why you see a role model as being someone in authority. Can't you learn from people who are not in authority?

Diane: It has to be someone in authority because we don't have a static work force so a role model is important.

A.S.: Diane, it seems to me that you see a role model as someone who has the authority to pass on the nursing culture of this unit. By this I mean that the role model in fact makes sure that the nursing staff know how things are done here in ICU.

Diane: Yes.

A.S.: Can you see problems in this way of thinking? You are in fact passing on what may be unexamined habits and procedures because of the fact that this is the accustomed way of acting in this ICU. Can you see that this could act against the development of thinking, creative nurses.

Diane: Yes, true. I will think about that while I check that dressing.

Later.

Diane: I think what I really mean is that the person who is in charge should be seen as a good example of a nurse and that other nursing staff will learn from her example. If someone asks me a question, I just jump in and show them. Do it with them.

A.S.:   Do all senior nurses provide a good role model for junior staff?

Diane: No way.

A.S.:   Then is learning about nursing necessarily related to authority or role models?

Diane: I guess I have never thought about that.

A.S.:   Then what are you doing when you teach by example, demonstration and discussion? Is what you do only appropriate when you have an authority role or do you do it at other times.

Diane: No, you are right. I act that way whether I am in charge or not. I like to help other nurses think about why they do things and sometimes I learn new ways of doing things from our discussions. I have to go and do this blood gas now so I will think about what I am really doing when I work with junior nurses.

          A few minutes later.

Diane: I've been thinking. It has to do with nursing knowledge. That's what has to be passed on.

A.S.:   What is nursing knowledge?

Diane: I am not sure. I have to think about that.

          Later.

Diane: I know that nursing knowledge is more than what we can learn about in books or lectures. I think that I mean the way in which nurses pass on knowledge about nursing.

A.S.:   Do you mean that knowledge that relates to nursing practice—to what you do as a practicing ICU nurse?

Diane: Yes, that's right.

    Phase 4.   I conducted an in-depth open-ended interview with each nurse to discuss their personal/professional nursing histories and examine the ways in which these histories had influenced their values, their nursing knowledge, and their nursing practices. By discussing the nurse's values, beliefs, and assumptions about nursing and the way in which these had evolved or been constructed over time, we were able to locate the development of power relations at work and the corresponding means of knowledge construction. These interviews were tape-recorded, and the transcripts were given back to the nurses.

Phase 5. A further in-depth interview was conducted with the nurse based on the transcripts. During this interview the nurses were able to raise issues from the transcript that they wanted to follow through, and I was able to raise areas that interested me. In this way we negotiated the content of the reflective process. This material was returned to the nurses for further comment.

Phase 6. During the final phase I developed a tentative theoretical framework for the description and analysis of nursing practice and talked it through with the four nurses remaining in the study.

Data Analysis Techniques

In an endeavor to develop a multifaceted perspective on the data, the material was triangulated in a number of ways.

Respondent Validation. The research participants had access to the research data and could comment on and correct it to the extent that I was mistaken in the medical/nursing details. This reflexive process enabled the nurses to reflect on their actions and practices. This reflection led at times to changes or attempted changes in their practices or to recognition that over time they perceived the issues differently. The fact that an ethnographic case study takes place over time enabled us to collect evidence of changes in attitudes and practices for analysis.

The validation by the research participants often occurred as a click of recognition, an "oh, yes" experience. The repetition of these experiences enabled us to place isolated instances of practice within a time frame in a specific social context.

Unlike an interpretive ethnography in which the intersubjective meanings would be the focus of the analysis, this critical ethnography used the intersubjective meanings as the basis for contestation and critique to uncover issues related to power/knowledge. Questions were posed such as: "Whose interests are being served in this practice?" and "How do those power relations affect the development of your nursing knowledge?"

Construct Validity. The data from the participant observation, the interviews, and other documents was examined to locate inferences and constructs for validation. These constructs were often then tested on other groups of nurses with whom I was associated through my work at the university and through my participation in another research project focusing on nursing practice as a basis for curriculum development. Although the nurses in this study did not keep regular professional journals, they all wrote a few isolated descriptions and reactions to their practice. These helped validate the material that I was gathering and the material that I had read in professional journals kept by other nurses engaged in nursing practice.

Field Relations: Impression Management; Field Roles and Managing Marginality

Impression Management. The hierarchical structure of the hospital identifies and demarcates its employees with clearly structured dress regulations. This caused me some initial concern as hospital security had been increased and the general reaction to any person who was not wearing some kind of uniform—including the stethoscope and/or badge, which constituted the uniform of some doctors, or the pyjamas/ nightie uniform of the patients—was to assume that they were either a patient, visitor, or unauthorized person. As the hospital was subject to its share of regular bomb hoaxes, minor fires, and thefts of valuables and drugs, staff were instructed to make inquiries of anyone who was not in uniform. I did not want to stand out and be constantly quizzed as to my intentions; yet it was not appropriate for me to wear a uniform, and the hospital would not provide me with an official hospital badge. After discussions with the nurse-researcher it was decided that I should wear a badge with my name followed by the words *Researcher, Deakin University.* I also noticed that no female staff member wore trousers, and on the first day I read a memo reminding all female staff that they were required to wear pantihose for reasons of infection control. The nursing uniform was white with a navy cardigan, so I decided to wear a dress or skirts blouses and jacket in similar colors to blend in somewhat. Nevertheless in the beginning, despite my badge, I still found myself being constantly asked if I required guidance or assistance. I decided that I would need to cultivate a manner of presentation that suggested that I belonged. This meant walking rapidly with my head held high looking straight ahead and appearing in control even when I would have preferred to take my time and actively peruse my surroundings and its inhabitants. This change in personal demeanor saved me from the constant inquiries given to outsiders and gave me access to general information about insider activities even from perfect strangers encountered in lifts.

Other insider-status activity in which I engaged when in the presence of unknown staff in a ward was making use of my permission to have access to rosters and nursing reports. I would sit down at the staff desk and read reports which immediately identified me as an insider as did the use of the staff phones. Another sign of insider status is the wearing of a motoroller (pager) or being voice-paged. Voice-paging is essential when the highly mobile hospital staff want to locate other staff members. The voice-page is not loud and can easily merge with all the other hospital noises. Outsiders ignore voice-paging, but insiders always listen. I was voice-paged on three occasions before I learned to listen, but I found that when I was introduced to other staff, some of them mentioned that they had heard my name over the voice-page and wondered who I was. I began to hear, and then recognize, new names over the voice-page, which was mostly used for regular staff.

The most interesting aspect of this impression management related to my badge. It was very different from the hospital staff badge; many staff would surreptitiously read the words *Researcher, Deakin University.* I then found that I would be addressed by doctors and sometimes paramedics but totally ignored by nurses and ancillary staff. Even when I explained to the medical staff that I was interested in nursing issues and not medical ones, I found that they would continue to talk to me about their work or stop and explain things to me in relation to medical conditions. After three days of this I changed my badge to read "Nursing Researcher, Deakin University." I was no longer specifically addressed by doctors who from then on tolerated my presence observing them at work with nurses or ignored me. However, I found myself being addressed by almost every nurse that I encountered anywhere in the hospital. A common question was "What is your research about?" followed by "Can I be in it?" Although I was unable to incorporate these nurses into my project as research informants/participants, I found that many of them would seek me out in break times to talk about my observations and give me their impressions and ideas about nursing issues. Some actively encouraged me to come and observe them when there was something typical or unusual in nursing procedures that I may not have seen before. This meant that I obtained access to other parts of the hospital, such as the operating suite, which would not have been possible otherwise. By these procedures I managed to make myself functionally invisible to those who would treat me as a visitor or unauthorized intruder and to those staff who were not interested in nursing research, while making myself visible to nurses.

Field Roles.   During the research I adopted the role of participant-observer. This role evolved differently over time. Initially my unfamiliarity with the setting and the social and professional roles operating there led me to suspend judgement and to document much descriptive data for later organization and analysis. As the settings and the nursing roles became familiar the observer role diminished in favor of a more participatory role. This participation could never be complete because I was not working in a discipline in which I was a practitioner. I would always need to engage with the research participants to develop meaningful interpretations of the data. However, as I chose to make this a reflexive engagement, my role began to be one of equal participant in the identification of issues and themes and reinterpretations of the data. This was interspersed with periods of time when I withdrew from the field site to allow time and space for reflection on the data and the jointly created meanings. The provision of the transcribed tapes of the joint discussions of the themes and issues in the data entailed some delay, which also enabled the participants to stand back from the motives and events of the moment and to reflect more analytically upon the data and the emerging theories. This disengagement from the data in order to analyze it turned us once again into observers of nursing practices.

Managing Marginality.   Despite the emphasis on the participatory nature of the data analysis, my status on the field site meant that I had to manage a position of marginality towards the research participants and the other members of the field site. According to Lofland (1971), the marginality of the simultaneous insider-outsider role enables the ethnographer to generate creative insight. For this creative insight to develop I had first to deal with my own stress and fears at the challenge of the task and the novelty of feeling useless in situations of crisis when everyone around me had set tasks and roles into which to retreat to disguise their own fears and feelings. The initial unfamiliarity of the setting when I did not have a role perceived by others to be functional and when I was concerned that I would not intrude on interpersonal intimacy between staff and patients or be "in the way" in emergencies or even routine treatments, added to my unease and feelings of marginality. Documentation of this unease proved to be useful in later discussions with staff as it alerted them more fully to the fears and anxieties experienced by patients, relatives, and friends and contributed to the adoption by these people of readily identifiable roles such as the "good patient," the "demanding relative," the "timid friend" and the particular behaviors associated with the adopted roles.

However, it also became apparent that my difficulties with maintaining the complexity of the marginal insider-outsider role was not as easily observed by others, and the feedback from the staff, patients,and visitors assured me that my strategies of impression management had succeeded in camouflaging me enough to make me appear as someone who "belonged," in the sense of being appropriate in the situation, even though my role there was not always clear to the uninitiated.

10

❦

Now You See Me, Now You Don't

The childhood game of hide and seek has much in common with the experience of nurses who work in busy clinical contexts. Their work is carried out under the public gaze, and yet their work is functionally invisible to many people, including their nursing colleagues. Foucault (1980a) argues that traditional forms of power meant that the power was manifest and visible to all through constant actions which display its potency, whereas in modern forms power becomes invisible while the objects of power become visible. He argues that this constant visibility of objects of power is constituted and maintained through hierarchical surveillance and is the key to the disciplinary technology of power. A superficial observation of a modern hospital, peopled by staff in differing uniforms representing different functions, readily demonstrates the hierarchical visibility of the objects of power relations. However, a closer examination uncovers a dialectic at work when the visible objects of power become invisible to others depending on the time, place, role, and the power relationship. This invisibility can adversely affect the access to knowledge and the capacity to engage in decision-making processes based around power relations.

Visibility: Uniforms as Technologies of Power/Knowledge

The clearest method of identifying people is to make them instantaneously recognizable by requiring them to wear a uniform. This hospital was no exception, and each person who

has a legitimate right to be there is required to be readily identifiable both as an insider and as to the function and status
that the person enjoys within the institution. The function of
the person's role is demonstrated by the kind of uniform they
are required to wear.

A. The patient uniform

The patient's uniform varies from personal pyjamas or
nighties to the impersonal hospital gowns and includes the
various stages of nudity that can be necessary in intensive
care. The patient's uniform identifies them as someone who is
functionally dependent on the services provided by the staff of
the hospital. The staff learn to feel comfortable with this kind
of distinction and can become uncomfortable with patients
who do not comply. Patients who are admitted for surgical procedures on the day prior to surgery may not feel sick and may
not feel like getting into bed in the middle of the afternoon.
As one nurse reported:

RN: I wish she would get into her nightie and get into bed.
She says that she feels well and hates being in bed,
especially at four in the afternoon, but even though I
know she is right she makes me uncomfortable.

A.S.: Why does she make you feel uncomfortable?

RN: I am used to looking around the ward and seeing if
everyone is alright and expecting to see them in bed. If
they are not, then I mentally think about where they are
in case they may need help such as with toileting...if I
see someone different in ordinary clothes sitting in a
chair by the bed, then I think they are a visitor. Then I
realize that she isn't and that she is my responsibility...Another thing is that I like to get my work finished
and when I look at her I think now that's something not
done yet (getting the female patient into her nightie and
into bed).

A.S.: Do you have to do something more for this patient at
the moment?

RN: No not really, I admitted her (took down the relevant
data) and took her obs (observations) while she sat in
the chair as she wouldn't get into bed. It is habit really.

> I am used to thinking that my work of admitting
> a patient is finished when they get into bed.

This nurse is used to understanding her role with the patient in terms of the patient's visibility to her. She identifies those over whom she has responsibility as people in night attire preferably situated in bed. In this situation the control of the patient is better effected not only through her visibility in a patient's uniform but by her relegation to a particular space, which is the hospital bed designated to her. The nurse feels comfortable with a docile patient who adopts a dependent patient role even when that role is not necessary or rationally defensible. A patient who violates this role by acting independently and sitting fully dressed in the visitor's chair challenges the nurse's right to make decisions for her when she is capable of making them for herself.

The nurse is also uncomfortable with the fact that the independent and rationally defensible position adopted by the patient also violates the nurse's need to have her in bed to demonstrate that her admitting task is completed. Here, the habits related to the task of admitting a patient conflict with the needs of the patient to maintain normality and independence until dependence becomes necessary. It is interesting that although this patient is quite visible in her difference to other patients she becomes momentarily invisible to the nurse in her routine assessment of the patients in the room. Her lack of patient uniform and her occupancy of the space used by visitors makes her "disappear" in her relation to the nurse, who then has to remind herself of her responsibility to this patient.

B. The ancillary staff uniform

The hospital had a large number of ancillary staff who were all required to wear uniforms, which identified their work roles and functions. For ease of hierarchical visibility each uniform was easily recognizable by its color and often its pattern. Some of these roles have been described by the color of the uniform such as the well-known "pinkies," a term used to identify cleaning ladies. These uniforms held important coded meaning for the hospital staff, which was beyond the investigative scope of this study. However, I was made aware of the fine distinctions when in my notes I identified a woman in a green uniform as a "cleaning lady" as she had been cleaning down a bed with disinfectant before being asked to help a nurse turn a patient. When the nurse saw my notes she said, "Oh that's wrong. She wasn't a cleaner, she was a nurse assistant."

C. The paramedic uniforms

The different paramedic groups had different uniforms, which identified their roles. Although for some, such as the physiotherapists, this was actually a distinct uniform, for others such as social workers, pharmacists, or dieticians the uniform was the white laboratory coat favored by the junior medical staff (and occasional senior medical staff).

D. The medical uniform

These uniforms varied from the white laboratory coat and stethoscope through to the badge, street clothes, and stethoscope of more senior medical staff. Some medical specialists used no other identifying signs than their sense of familiarity and "presence" on the ward or their retinue of junior medical staff. Although the medical staff were presented with identification badges, many did not bother wearing them. Nurses claimed that this wasted the time of personnel who needed to identify medical staff and differentiate them from the hospital visitors. They reported that when cases of mistaken identity occurred it sometimes caused further difficulties with some medical staff who expected the nursing staff to recognize them.

Uniforms for nurses were usually argued on grounds of hygiene and infection control. It was apparent that this argument did not hold for medical staff who often had close contact with a number of patients in succession, even in intensive care, but who were not required to do more than wash their hands between patients. This point was not lost on nurses who wondered if it was possible that only nurses are able to spread germs, as evident from my notes collected on Bev on 8 August 1987.

Today Bev asked me to put on a disposable plastic apron whenever I entered her bay. Her patient had just returned from heart bypass surgery and she was stabilizing him. I readily agreed to her request. However, when I left the bay I noticed that the doctors were having close contact with the patient without donning protective clothing. I mentioned this to Bev, and she said sarcastically:

Don't you know...doctors don't have germs!...look at that doctor now bending over that patient who has just had open heart surgery. See how his tie is dragging over the patient's chest area. Next he will go and lean over another patient, and another, and his tie will trail all over them...but it doesn't matter because his tie doesn't have germs!

E. The nurse uniform

All nurses working on the wards wore uniforms. The nurse educators, nurse-researcher, and nurse administrators wore badges and street clothes although when on the wards they sometimes wore the white laboratory coat of the medical staff, an interesting status correlation. The clinical nurses were therefore readily identifiable to other staff by their uniforms although the uniforms differed with seniority and status. The nursing supervisors wore white uniforms with long sleeves, whereas the graduate nurses wore similar uniforms with short sleeves. The student nurses being trained at the hospital wore colored uniforms with status indicators of their seniority and these differed in color and style from those worn by the student nurses from the college diploma course. State Enrolled Nurses (SENs) were similarly identifiable.

Nursing Uniforms: Nursing Visibility

These distinctive uniforms made each particular nurse visible to other staff members, a process that facilitates control. Nurses could readily be identified as being in the wrong place or as being in the right place at the wrong time because the routines and movements of each role were known to their superiors. Nurses could readily be identified by doctors, patients, or other staff who wanted their attention, although it was not always easy for these people to identify which kind of nurse they needed. Therefore, student nurses would receive requests from patients which needed to be directed to the nurse in charge, and charge nurses would be asked for things that would be the responsibility of a more junior nurse. Eve, a charge nurse who moved to become a charge nurse at another hospital, found that her new charge nurse uniform had distinguishing shoulder tabs to identify her as the charge nurse. This heightened her visibility in the hospital to those who rec-

ognized the symbolic authority invested in the tabs although
this was not apparent to the patients or their relatives.

The regulations concerning the correct nursing uniform
are directed by senior staff and justified on grounds of hygiene
and discipline. The charge nurses are required to ensure that
their nurses and ancillary staff are correctly attired in regulation uniform. Although the nurses in the study did not object
to wearing some kind of uniform, they did object to the regulation of the uniform and the need for this to be policed by other
staff rather than allowing individual nurses to take responsibility for dressing appropriately. When challenged the nurses
agreed that they had accepted the wearing of uniforms
because that had always been part of nursing and most mentioned that they were practical to wash. Further discussions
suggested that the requirement of a regulation uniform for
nurses demonstrates an area in which nurses are subject to
oppressive administrative practices that are not consistent
with the requirements made of other health workers. Nursing
discipline means that the charge nurses are then required to
police their own oppression as well as the oppression of their
staff because they are required to support and maintain hospital uniform requirements.

The visibility of a uniform enables the nurse to become visible in the hierarchical hospital system and reflects the power
relations at work. In the same way a uniformed nurse was privy
to particular kinds of knowledge about particular patients and
their families. This knowledge extended beyond the scope of
medical data to include socioeconomic, psychological, familial,
and various other aspects relating to the person who had
become a "patient." This knowledge is acquired both formally
and informally by nurses in the conduct of their clinical work.
Some of the knowledge is volunteered by the patient, either in
deference to the authority vested in the nursing uniform or in
response to the good clinical skills of the nurse. The nurse also
has access to other information in the patient's files, which the
patient does not have access to and which if they did, they
might not want disseminated. However, the uniformed nurse
has only limited access to all the information in the hospital,
and by virtue of the visibility of the uniform a nurse can be
readily identified as being in the wrong place, such as attending
a clinical medical meeting uninvited. As one nurse commented
when she left the staff room at the end of her tea break:

Wouldn't it be great to just stay on and discuss a patient problem with the doctors like that social worker and occupational therapist are doing. But duty calls for nurses and so all of us in nursing uniforms have to get up and leave. (RN)

Nursing Uniforms: Nursing Invisibility

The apparent visibility accorded by a nursing uniform also serves to make nurses invisible as distinct individuals with specific role, function, knowledge, and expertise within the wider group of people designated as nurses. Nurses suggested that this kind of invisibility is selective depending on the people with whom they are involved.

Carol: ...I think that you are invisible to the doctors when you are a new graduate. I know when I started training we were taught to treat the doctor like a god. Some of them still think that they are God and you are their servants. Some of them use you all the time but don't think that you know much at all. Now the doctors have to treat me properly because I am in charge. I get on alright with most of them because they know me and I can say what I want. I don't think that they know many of the nurses. I think anyone dressed in a white uniform becomes invisible to some of them until they want something done.

After an experience of being ignored by a new social worker and then a medical student at the front desk a senior nurse said:

Do I look invisible to you? I would have thought that I could be easily seen. I take up enough space. Some people are amazing. They don't seem to see nurses at all. No one introduces themselves, and you have to peer at their badges. But many of the doctors and paramedics don't bother wearing their badges, and no one knows who they are. It is not so bad for me because I have been here a long time and I know most of the regular staff...and I'm not scared to ask them who they are, but it is confusing for some of the other nursing staff if they ask them questions. You don't know if you are talking to a doctor, a social worker or what. They often don't tell us what they are doing or ask us questions, which is crazy because we are the ones who are here all the time. (RN)

I enjoyed wearing street clothes during the strike, and it was amazing how many doctors and paramedics spoke to me who don't usually. They certainly take more notice of you when you are dressed in street clothes like them. When they see you coming, they have to look carefully to see who you are, whereas when you are in uniform they see the white clothes coming and ignore you. However, I think it is better for the patients to have a nurse in uniform. They know who to speak to when they need help, especially the older patients who can be confused by the number of people around them. (Charge nurse, geriatric ward)

This indicates a process of selective visibility in medical and paramedical staff who tend to pay attention to particular nurses such as charge and associate charge nurses and ignore other nurses until such time as they particularly need the help of a particular nurse. The data contains numerous examples of this selective visibility and the dependence of medical staff on the senior nurse, but one incident from my notes was particularly telling.

When I arrived Carol was just telling the specialist who had been very involved with her on the ward that she was leaving to take charge of another ward.

He responded with "Oh...who will take over?"

Carol explained that the charge position would be advertised but that—(the next senior nurse on the ward) would be the acting charge nurse until a new charge nurse was appointed.

The specialist asked: "Who's she?"

Carol told me that she was amazed because this nurse was always acting in-charge on the days when she wasn't working a day shift, and this specialist had worked with this particular nurse on ward rounds for years. However, later reflecting on this incident Carol suggested that she "shouldn't have been amazed as this particular specialist has poor interpersonal skills."

Patient Invisibility

Another constant theme in the data was the apparent invisibility of the patients to many doctors and some nurses—even to those who were treating them. This invisibility begins with the medical focus on the system or the part of the body under treatment, which reduces the patient to "the hernia in bed 2" or "the CAGS patient in bay 6." This description of a person as an illness denies the interrelationship of the whole person with their illness, their family and friends, and with their community. This process can lead to a another dimension of patient invisibility reported by nurses, when the medical data about the patient becomes more important in diagnosis and treatment than the patient themselves or the knowledge about the patient acquired by the nurse in the process of nursing them.

Eve reports:

I have seen doctors come into the bay and ignore the patient in the bed and focus on the information in the charts and make a decision about the patient just based on that. There is a big difference in what is in the charted information and what can be observed in the patient. Doctors miss lots by ignoring the patient and the information that they can get from the nurse who has been at the bedside all day.

Many nurses echoed this frustration when medical staff entered the ward or bay where they were working and ignored both them and the patients, making decisions based on their assessments of the data in the charts. In situations where the patient information is not kept at the bedside the doctors may not even visit the patient, relying entirely on their judgement of the data collected by the nurse and the information acquired through the technological interventions. Therefore, medical and scientific knowledge is legitimated as superior to subjective observation, intuition, and the skilled practical knowledge acquired over time by the nurse. As a consequence of this kind of medical action nurses reported many instances of the inappropriate treatments being ordered for the "invisible" patient.

Eve describes the danger to a female patient when the doctors relied on the charted information and their knowledge:

We had a lady here who had been in 5 weeks with renal failure. She was on dialysis and when she was taken off she bled profusely. The resident was told, and he ordered a drug but did not go and assess what the drug had done. When it came to the ward round with the specialist the resident hurriedly gave him the information from the chart and they made a decision to prescribe another drug from that information. I was standing with them outside the bay, and as I looked at the patient I could see that she had just had a stroke. I knew that if they gave the patient that particular drug it would be extremely dangerous in her present condition. They would have known, too, if they had stopped for one moment and looked at the patient instead of the charts. The charts did not show what had just happened (the stroke) and how that changed everything.

They were busy talking among themselves, and I guess I put myself down because instead of challenging them about their choice of the drug for the present state of the patient I just said:

I think her conscious state is much worse.

The resident responded by quoting the information on the charts, so then I said:

I think she has had a stroke.

They then had a look at the woman and finally agreed that she had suffered a stroke. I then argued that the proposed treatment would be contraindicated, and eventually they changed the orders.

In this situation the data was accorded more authority by the doctors than the observations of the nurse. The experience of being treated as invisible in the diagnostic process made it very difficult for even this senior nurse to demonstrate the value of her practical nursing knowledge. Instead she engaged in the doctor/nurse game in an endeavor to help the doctors discover the problem for themselves ("I think her conscious state is much worse."), and so maintained the superiority of their objective knowledge over her subjective knowledge gained through extensive skilled clinical observations. In this instance as the doctors did not participate in the doctor/nurse game, she was forced to give them her own diagnosis from her observation of the patient ("I think she has had a stroke."). Although Eve was sure that the patient had suffered a stroke, she still put forward her diagnosis in a tentative form rather than making a statement as she would have done with her nursing peers. This example demonstrates the manner in which the oppressive power relations of medical domination are mirrored in the oppression of nursing knowledge. The nurse becomes invisible as a participant in the diagnostic process in the same way as practical nursing knowledge becomes invisible to the doctor who judges it against the visibility of the technical data.

Visibility: The Public Nature of the Workplace

Nursing is practiced in the public sphere. Nursing actions are generally carried out in places where they are open to public scrutiny from a wide variety of people with different knowledge, expectations, and understandings of the nature of clinical nursing practice. Working under public scrutiny is not unique to nursing, all the hospital ancillary and clinical staff work in situations where they are generally observable. This public scrutiny may not be as big a problem for ancillary staff who are engaged in tasks such as cleaning and serving meals, but it can be very problematic for doctors, paramedics, and nursing staff. The medical and paramedical staff generally spend only a portion of their working day on the wards under public scrutiny, but nurses need to learn to work in cramped spaces under the gaze of interested staff, families, and relatives. An excerpt from my notes describes the number and variety of staff and other people occupied on a medical ward at late morning.

11:55 a.m.   An orthopedic specialist arrived and wanted to discuss a patient with Carol. As the ward felt considerably busy and crowded, I decided to make a count of the number of staff on the ward. As there were two doctor's rounds in progress, there was a total of sixteen doctors and medical students visiting the ward. There was the aforementioned orthopedic specialist, the Charge Nurse (Carol), two RN's, two SENs, one ward clerk, two nursing assistants, two cleaners, two women delivering

meals, one dietician, two physiotherapists, one
college tutor, two college students, one clinical
nurse teacher supervising an overseas trained
nurse, and myself. This totaled thirty-six staff,
including students, myself (making thirty-seven),
three relatives and twenty-one patients, a total of
sixty-one people sitting, standing, or lying down
in one small ward.

The ability to cope with this public scrutiny is part of the
nurse's socialization to the nursing role. In discussions experienced staff did not raise this as an issue as it had become a
taken-for-granted aspect of their nursing practice, but new
graduates talked about this as a problem both to me and in
front of me on a number of occasions.

During the tea break Carol suggested that we go and have
morning tea with a nurse who was a new graduate...the
nurse confessed that she wished that she was invisible
until she got more confidence on the ward. I asked her if
she was anxious, and she said:

I am scared stiff all the time. There is so much to remember and its so easy to make mistakes.

Carol assured her that this was normal for new nurses
and that she would feel much better soon. The RN then
told us how she was terrified of doctors and sure that she
was going to make a mistake in front of them. Carol said:

I am not afraid of them. If I don't agree, I just tell them.
(Carol, C.N, medical ward)

This new graduate was still very aware of her visibility in front
of others, particularly doctors, whereas Carol who is a very
experienced senior nurse, has confidence in her clinical judgement and her clinical practice. During further discussion Carol
assured the new graduate that she had experienced the same
feelings when she began nursing and that it took time to get
used to working under public scrutiny. Other nurses in the
study spoke of the need to keep junior nurses under constant
observation in order to help them learn and to minimize the
consequences of mistakes.

11:20 a.m.   Eve checks on a nurse who has had the curtains pulled around her bay for most of the morning.

Eve (to me):   This girl is a junior nurse, and she keeps pulling the curtains around. It worries me as she doesn't want anyone to see her doing tasks. It's scary—especially when she has a junior medico in there, too! If she left the curtains open she would get more help and support. This way I keep wanting to check up on her all the time. I see the curtains closed, and when I know that there is no big procedure due I naturally think there might be a problem. I go in to see if she is OK, and she is doing blood gases or something basic like that (Eve, CN, ICU).

Eve is concerned that this nurse needs to learn to work under scrutiny so that the more experienced nurses can provide help and support. This is consistent with Eve's emphasis on the teaching element of the senior nurse's role. Discussions with the nurse in question indicated that she was not concerned about observation by senior nursing staff in the unit but by medical staff, paramedics, and the patient's visitors. Therefore, avoidance of public scrutiny can serve to isolate the nurse from nursing peers and reduce the possibility for constructive feedback.

Diane: I am pretty much a loner so I don't get the same feedback from the peer group as other nurses.

A.S.:   I wonder if that is true of nurses. It appears to me from my discussions that a lot of nurses feel isolated and inadequate about themselves and have low self-esteem and often...you can notice the negative things in others rather than the positive, or if you do notice the positive it only makes you feel more inadequate.

Diane: Yes. Positive reinforcement is something I am very aware of and I always try to (do)—especially now that I have got a more senior position. I went up to a girl the other day, and she is the real cream of nursing; she is just fabulous, only a new grad. She is only in her first year out and working on ICU. I was in charge that day, and I wasn't sure how long she was staying in ICU because I knew that she had come from one of the wards where we send our patients to, and so I said to her: "Are you just down here for three months and then going back up to the ward where you have been?" And she just said: "Oh no I am going to another hospital to do the intensive care course in August, and I will probably be here till then." I said: "Oh we are going to lose you; that's a shame." She said: "Do you really mean that?" I said: "Of course, you have been terrific. You have worked really well; you have picked up really quickly; you are a joy to teach." She stood there and then she just burst into tears. I said, "what's the matter?" and she said, "I really needed that today. I have been feeling so stupid, and I am not picking up, and I am not doing things right."

...Everyone (in the ward) had been saying "isn't this girl fantastic" and yet no one had said it to her. She had just had no positive reinforcement because everyone assumed she knew that she was always fantastic, and she is obviously a perfectionist, too, that (sic) demands a lot of herself. So I rounded up the clinical teachers and said, "listen you have got to do something, you have got to tell this girl she is alright." ...I am conscious of it (the need for positive feedback), so I make a point of doing it if I can. Yes, there is not much of it in nursing. You always get criticized before you get praised.

This incident highlights the visibility dialectic for nurses. Feelings of inadequacy, which flow from trying to cope with the pressure of constant observation from other staff members, can lead nurses to keep themselves separate from other nurses and in a sense to learn to act as if they were invisible. Nurses learning to act as if their work was invisible to others soon learn to act as if other nurse's work is invisible to them. This causes difficulties in the development of clinical knowledge because nurses are not encouraged to collaborate or to provide adequate support and feedback to each other. This symbolic invisibility of nurse's actions to each other also causes problems when a nurse is required to make an assessment of another nurse as Diane found when she was acting in charge of the ICU unit.

D: Being in the Charge nurse job for the last two months there were a number of assessments that were due and had to be done. I had virtually no experience writing assessments prior to taking on this job, and I found writing assessments was enormously difficult because it made me reassess the quality of my supervision of my staff. I would find that I had a general idea of how someone worked and a general feeling attached to that about that person's qualities, but when I had to actually itemize it, for some people, I found it quite impossible. For some people I would have to go and canvass all the senior staff in the unit to get a more coherent picture. For a few assessments it took me a couple of weeks to have on the back burner in my mind before I could actually write those. It made me just sit back and look at my job description and say what I am doing is not what is really required of me, which is a problem because the associate charge nurse role is a new role and is obviously going to go through a few stages of development. It certainly brought home the responsibilities of the role to me. But coming back to writing assessments. The assessment form that we use at the hospital is one of the better ones that I have seen out of an awfully bad lot. There is no structured interview process for people as they go along in their work so when they get their assessment, that's it. If it is good, then that's fine, but if it is bad, then it can be quite devastating. Also, I find that nurses find it hard to give positive feedback. I can do that, but I am almost incapable of giving negative feedback to people and that's a skill to be learned, and there is no formal training at all available to us in these kind of skills.

This meant that two of the junior staff were up for assessment and everybody knew that they weren't up to scratch. I had people knocking on my door saying, "what are you going to do. I can't stand it anymore. I can't cope." When it came to their assessment they both resigned after they had been given their assessments which made me feel (sarcastically) fantastic! One of the girls I had known personally through my union work and I actually recommended that she come to the unit. I had seen her being self-directed, take responsibility; she had quite a good analytical mind, but in ICU all that didn't seem to apply. She wasn't able to transfer those skills and use them in that area. It had been a very difficult problem. I didn't want to give her an assessment because I knew her personally and was quite fond of her, but no one else wanted to do it. But one nurse agreed to do it (for me) because I knew her. I wrote up a a rough assessment because the hardest part is getting the words on the paper. I gave it to the other associate charge and said, "this is the impression I have from everyone else, feel free to change it at will." So she and another associate charge presented this (the assessment), and the girl was quite distraught and didn't come to work the next time she was on duty.Then she called me up, and I spent a long time talking to her about the appraisal and her reaction to it, and she used quite a lot of emotional manipulation in the way she spoke. She said the whole process stank, and the way it was delivered stank, and the way that she was left alone in the room as she had asked to be stank, and all sorts of things. Because I had become extremely aware of how bad the process was myself, I couldn't disagree. I found it very difficult to pull her up and say you are using emotional manipulation here and not accepting responsibility for your poor performance. I couldn't say that to her because I knew that she had not been pre-pared in a structured way so that she could expect that kind of assessment when she got it. All the senior staff had said to me, "she has had far more input than any-body else. She doesn't really take responsibility for patients; she is always coming to us for reinforcement, and we have to be always checking up on her. She has had far more personal tutes than anyone else on equip-ment, and she is still not making the grade." We all knew for someone to be requiring all that they obviously were not making the grade, but to her that was what she expected people to do for her. She wasn't thinking that this was anything out of the ordinary.

A.S.:   Do you mean that she didn't understand the standards of practice that she had to meet and that she wasn't meeting them?

D: Yes, they are not laid down or told along the way. I guess you are just supposed to pick them up. But she didn't, and she didn't know that she wasn't performing well. That's why she was so angry when she found out. She just resigned and went and worked in a nursing home. That was horrible experience for me because I was the one who felt guilt.

Through this reflection on her clinical practice, Diane is able to recognize that when she was required to write assessments on the practice of others she had very little idea of how they were working. Their nursing practice had become functionally invisible to her despite the fact that her role as associate charge nurse required her to move in and out of the bays providing support to the nurses working in the unit. As is evident from the discussion reported earlier in this section, Diane is in fact able to recognize good clinical practice and to provide positive feedback. My written observations of Diane's work demonstrate her ability to foresee potential difficulties for staff and to provide effective interventions. In circumstances such as these the clinical practice of her nurses is very visible to her.

Selective Visibility

It appears that Diane and the other nurses demonstrated a process of selective visibility towards other nurses' nursing practices. When they were aware of potential problems for other nurses, they would keep an eye on the nurse in question for the duration of the potential difficulty but then they would ignore that nurse's work. These potential difficulties generally occurred when the nurse was to be involved in a particularly difficult or unpleasant technique, or needed to cope with new technology, or when the patient or family were causing emotional problems. Nurses may also ask for help in these situations, but they rarely discuss or ask for help in their regular clinical practices. On the medical ward nurses asked for help to get tasks completed or discussed patients or doctors, but again it was very evident that, as a survival strategy, the nurses had opted to focus on their own work, ignoring the public scrutiny of their work by others and ignoring the clinical practice of others. This was particularly evident in relation to the general standard of clinical practice, which appeared invisible to the nurses, whereas very good practice was recognized and very poor practice was commented on. The stress of public scrutiny reported on by new graduates is soon replaced by a capacity to engage in this game of selective visibility. The game is thwarted when the RN becomes senior enough to be in charge of other nurses and to be required to assess them. Assessment then becomes an inspectorial process of examining the work of their peers rather than an ongoing process in which self-reflection and collaborative reflection informs the process. As Diane discovered when she was in the position of assessing other nurses, the experience of being judged against a standard that is never made explicit, in a culture full of unspoken values about clinical practice, which are never disclosed, by peers who have given no feedback on your skills and knowledge, is an experience of oppression and injustice. Nurses are disempowered by the culture of the ward, which adheres to implicit values and unexamined practices. According to Diane, the consequence of this disempowering process is the inability of staff to provide negative feedback in a constructive manner. Negative feedback becomes focused on the individual's inability to meet the implicit standards and ignores the structured inequities, which have contributed to the perceived unsatisfactory standard of clinical practice. This dialectic of selective visibility under public scrutiny also contributes to the feelings of isolation expressed by all nurses in the face of human suffering, which appears unjust and irrational.

Diane: I feel that when nursing staff are faced with difficult or painful incidents they cope with as much as they can for a certain length of time and then they withdraw or they don't cope. Then coming out from that I feel that their immediate superiors, whether it be the associate charge, charge nurse, or nursing supervisor, are people who should have the skills to recognize that an incident is occurring or has occurred, and then have the ability to recognize the effect that it has on the individual and the ability to help that individual if help is needed. I don't think any of the senior nursing staff that I have ever dealt with, or worked with, have ever had any of that sort of training. Some people have an inherent ability that they have developed through trial and error, but they don't have any training in that field at all and it is so important.

Diane's comments highlight the fact that the process of learning to cope with constant and obvious surveillance has led to a number of coping strategies. One of the most common is to focus on the task and attempt to finish it as quickly as possible in order to move away from the scrutiny. Nurses who work on task-based systems of patient allocation learn to move rapidly from patient to patient completing particular tasks such as medications or observations (temperature, pulse and blood pressure). Even in settings where the nurse is caring full time for only one patient, as in critical care areas or primary patient allocation, it is possible for nurses to structure their routine around the completion of tasks or to structure their tasks into times when they are less likely to be observed.

Visibility: Data Collection and Records

Foucault (1975) argues that technologies of power rely on close surveillance of the individuals within their walls. In hospitals patients are not only known through their physical bodies but are also known in the records kept on them. The data for these records are generally collected by nurses but include doctor's orders, programs of treatment devised by associated paramedics, and information obtained through technological means. Nurses are generally the keepers of the record by which the patient is known. These records enable the patient to be labeled and treated in specific ways. They enable hospital staff to engage in normalizing technologies by providing the data whereby the staff judge the amount of deviation from the norm for a "healthy, functioning body" and adapt strategies of remediation to remove the deviant body from its position of ill health to a position of health.

This recordkeeping task makes the patient both visible and invisible to the staff. Despite the oft-heard myth that "nurses never write," from my observations it was apparent that nurses write both regularly and often although much of what they write consists of the documentation for other people—medical staff, paramedics, and senior administrative staff. According to Foucault, this recordkeeping makes the patient visible and open to normalizing techniques. Evidence from my research indicates that the patient as a person can also become invisible in the record because of the inadequacy of the record-keeping processes. This occurs because nurses both deny themselves and are structurally denied the opportunity to engage in written language about clinical nursing practice. This is quite distinct from the ability of nurses to use technical and idiosyncratic language to describe medical and nursing procedures, patient health status, equipment use, and drug regimes.

Benner (1984:1) argues that nurses have not been careful recordkeepers of their own clinical learning. My own observations and discussions would support this statement. None of the clinical nurses involved in the research kept any regular record of their clinical practice other than what was routinely required of them by others. These records were not initiated and owned by the nurses and so do not contain the kind of information that would enable the nurses to examine their own nursing knowledge and practice.

Nursing Documentation

The kinds of recordkeeping that I have observed nurses engaging in can be categorized in the following ways:

A. Data for doctors

The first and most common form of recordkeeping is the collection of data for the use of the medical staff. This data is quantitative and often presented in chart form for easy accessibility. Although this kind of data may readily identify conditions, such as a high temperature in a patient, it does not document any evaluation of the cause or effect for the particular patient. The qualitative judgements about the quantitative information are generally not recorded. Therefore, the qualitative judgement that this patient has a history of higher than usual temperatures during illness is not recorded although it may be known to the nurses.

This kind of quantitative documentation is sometimes used by the nurse but is primarily available for the information of the assorted medical staff associated with the patient. The nurse, who is constantly with the patient, knows when there are changes in the patient's condition and the possible causes of the changes. Expert nurses use a combination of knowledge, skill, and experience, which they often call "gut feeling," which is similar to Polyani's (1962) concept of "connoisseurship," to predict changes in the conditions of patient before they are apparent or recordable. They also pass on that information to other nurses orally, either informally or through the procedure of a formal handover to the charge nurse and to the nurses on the next shift. The good nurse then checks the charted information against the oral report and their own assessment of the patient. Some nurses report this information to the medical staff, who also check all the written records, and others leave the staff to read the information for themselves.

One nurse told me:

> We collect all this information for the doctors, and they just come and look at the data to make their judgements. They don't ask the nurse who has been there (at the bedside) all day, what is happening with the patient. Some doctors hardly look at the patient; they make up their mind from the data. But the data doesn't give the whole picture by itself because each patient is different. You need to take note of other observations like their color or how responsive they are to stimuli like light or pressure.

Therefore, this kind of tacit knowledge about the patient can be lost for want of a structure by which to communicate it or an interested audience to receive and use the clinical knowledge. Despite the reliance of the medical staff on the data collected by the nurses, any discussions between them are oral, and the only kinds of records kept by the nurses are those pertaining to doctor's orders. The information supplied by the nurse, which has been used by the medical staff to inform their decisions concerning the patient, is unacknowledged in the written form. The decision consists of a one-line diagnosis and appropriate treatment or drug orders. The nurse becomes invisible in the diagnostic process because the written records do not detail the processes by which decisions have been reached and so does not acknowledge the nursing input.

Nurses participating in the research study reported that they believed that few nurses looked at the charted information and asked themselves what the information meant in the

way that the medical staff did. Nurses relied on the oral
reports from their nursing colleagues and on their own clinical
judgement to provide them with the kind of information that
was useful for their clinical decision making. This practice of
keeping information for others is also found in the requirements of data collection by various members of nursing administration. Unlike the data collected for doctors, which is collected by all nurses, the task of collecting and preparing data
required by administration falls more heavily on the senior
members of the nursing staff.

B. Data for nursing colleagues

The second major category of documentation is the collection of data by nurses for the use of their nursing colleagues.
This category would include nursing notes and the nursing
process. The inability of nurses to cooperate in writing effective
nursing care plans based on their clinical care is the bane of
many educators and administrators. They find that nurses
tend to copy out the quantifiable data already recorded on the
chart rather than passing on details about the kind of nursing
care being provided and making reasoned projections about
future care. In this way nursing care plans will contain facts
such as blood pressure and temperature and omit details such
as the fact that the patient was able to sit in a chair or was
very anxious after the visit of a particular relative.

In discussing the care plans Ann reported that many
nurses made sure that they didn't have time to write them during a shift. Although she does write them, it is obvious from
my notes that she is not filling them in appropriately.

During one shift as she filled in the notes she told me:

This is the worst bit...writing all this up. You have to write
out the same things over and over on different charts. See
I have to write this here...and here...and now again here. I
hate it...its so boring. I don't know why once isn't enough
but apparently they want to keep the records in this size
and the bedside charts are too large...or so they say. Then
we have to waste time writing up the nursing care plans.
We say it all again in handover and it is all on the charts.

Eve, in her role as charge nurse, was attempting to improve
the quality of the material in the nursing care plans.

11:05 a.m.   Eve spoke to a nurse who was writing up her nursing care plan while her patient slept.

Eve: Do you understand what you have to do with a care plan?

Nurse: Well, I understand some but not all. I think we write about patient management.

Eve: All right, let's see what you have here. Look this information is on his chart for the physio and is not related to his nursing care. Can you see any other problems with what has been written about this patient in the last four shifts?

Nurse: Well, there is nothing on here that tells us precisely what is wrong with the patient.

Eve: No, but that doesn't need to be here. That's irrelevant here. It's not a problem. That's not needed in a nursing care plan. We have all the information about that on his medical charts. A nursing care plan is for the nurse. It is supposed to tell you what care has been provided and what is needed.

Nurse: How do you mean?

Eve: If you looked at this plan you would have no idea from this whether the patient has been awake or asleep, whether he is sitting out of bed and for how long, or how his dressings were done. We don't know from this what special nursing care he has had, how he responded and what special nursing care he needs. What can we find out from this care plan?

Nurse: His temp, blood pressure, blood gases, respiratory rate, etc.

Eve: Yes, but all that information is on his medical charts so why spend time copying it out again?

Nurse: I thought that was what we should do.

Eve: Look this is where you are at, you are collecting all the medical things. Let's look at some other care plans and see if we can find out information about nursing care from them.

Nurse: What about this?

Eve: Yes, but what does it mean. It is very vague. The
                information needs to be put in accurate terms. Use
                your technical language and explain why/how etc.
                the nursing care was developed. Any nurse should
                be able to to read this and see what has happened
                with the patient and what is needed.

Later.

12:05 p.m.:   Eve was called by the nurse with whom she had
                been working on the nursing care plans. The
                nurse asked Eve to check what she had done. Eve
                told her that the content was greatly improved but
                that it was very confusing to read as the nurse
                had listed the changes that occurred over ten
                shifts in one column. This meant that the care
                plan read as if the patient had received fourteen
                changes of dressing in one shift.

This exchange demonstrates a common problem. Nurses
are not capturing on paper a picture of the patient and their
interactions with the nurse as a basis for further critical thinking, or theorizing, about the patient and their own clinical
practice. The effects of irregular and insufficient recordkeeping
is incomplete information about the patient, which is often
misleading. This is particularly apparent when nurses support
the technical data with their own interpretations of the data
without demonstrating that it is an interpretation, or indeed
making the effort to check out the data for reliability.

Carol: Nurses have a great difficulty writing. They write about
                their feelings and not about the facts. I have found it
                difficult to get nurses to write histories that describe
                the facts and not just an interpretation of them. For
                example, if a nurse comes into a room and finds a
                patient on the floor they will write in the patient's his-
                tory "fell out of bed." I will say "Did you see the patient
                fall?" "No, but I found them on the floor." "But you
                didn't see them fall out of bed?" "No." "Then write what
                you saw. Then we can find out what happened—if the
                patient fell, was pushed, got out themselves for some
                reason etc..." Nurses don't write reports accurately;

they write their interpretations. I think that there is a place for feelings in reports, but what we usually get is the nurse's interpretation, not the patient's feelings or interpretations.

Carol has highlighted a problem that is apparent when reading nursing notes. The notes rarely reflect the patient's view of the world with a carefully articulated picture of the clinical care that has been provided and the plans for future clinical care. Therefore, despite documentation, the patient as a whole person remains invisible as does the clinical nursing care being provided.

My observations of, and discussions with, clinical nurses would support Perry's (1985a) claim that many nurses regard recordkeeping as irrelevant. The difficulties of acquiring this kind of documentation are not only an area of constant concern for educators and administrators alike but a cause of annoyance to many RNs who see this kind of activity as a waste of time. Nurses passively resist and subvert procedures that are instituted to enable them to record their nursing practice on nursing notes and to make forecasts about the needs of particular patients. Nurses report that they rarely read the nursing notes, and it is never seen as a priority because the information contained in them often mirrors the information contained in the charts. I have asked nurses questions that have arisen directly from my reading of the nursing notes about a patient and have received replies such as:

Oh I haven't looked at them...we hear about the patients in handover.(RN, ICU)

or

I don't bother because they don't tell you things that you haven't heard at handover or can see for yourself from the charts and the patient.(RN, medical ward)

Despite support and encouragement from middle management and from educators, the nurses I observed did not really make an effort to improve their recording skills in what they regarded as a pointless exercise. The written word is not deemed necessary as it is rarely read carefully and is viewed only as a very inadequate representation of the clinical knowledge about the patient which is passed on orally. The written record is never expected to be an adequate substitute for the complexity and immediacy of the oral handover. The concerns, expressed by administrative staff and educators, that vital information can be lost in the oral handover was born out during one observation session when a nurse responded to a question based on the nursing notes with: "How did you know that? No one told me."

When I explained that I had read it in the nursing notes, the nurse replied that she had glanced at them but had missed that information. As the information was important she then acted on it. However, the attitudes of the nurses to the writing up of accurate and useful nursing notes was so negative that this was an isolated incident. It was the only time that I found that the notes actually contained some important information that had not been passed on orally. This was not an indication of a high standard of oral handover. Indeed, they seemed to vary from mediocre to excellent.

The following quote is more indicative of the attitude of the nurses to the writing up of nursing notes.

I am just writing up the nursing notes before I go. You only have to write one or two sentences about the patient. I don't know why we bother sometimes because we are told all the information in handover, and I am sure no one else but you reads them. Anyway, it is the same as in the charts (RN, ICU).

In this situation I was seen as needing to read them because I have only limited comprehension of the data collected in the charts.

C. Data for nursing practice

The third category of documentation kept by nurses and relating to patient care that I have observed was the kind of information that was instigated and used by nurses themselves. This information met a particular and immediate need. An example that I observed was the development by an RN of a chart to check on continent and incontinent patients in the geriatric assessment ward during the evening shift. This continence chart was designed by a staff member on night shift to collect the kind of necessary information for the planning of quality nursing care and for the assessment process. This documentation focused on only one aspect of patient care and was effective because it enabled the nurses to plan appropriate supports for incontinent patients. In this example a particular aspect of the patient became visible to the gaze of the recordkeepers.

In another observation a charge nurse documented the staffing and equipment needs, from a nursing perspective, which would be necessary for the unit if a complex new medical procedure was to be instigated in the hospital. Although this documentation was intended to demonstrate that quality patient care was at risk unless staffing and equipment needs were addressed, the documentation itself consisted of equipment lists, which the nurse used to back up her oral presentation. The nurse gave the doctor the information in the way in which he was used to receiving it from a nurse—an oral argument supported by brief written list. In contrast the doctor organized a staff meeting and presented his information in a talk with slides showing how patients would benefit from the operation. Through listening to the arguments on both sides, it was apparent that the doctor was particularly interested in the actual surgery and the opportunity to be the first Victorian doctor to do it, whereas the nurse was concerned with using her clinical knowledge to ensure the provision of quality patient care. However, the documentation provided by the doctor and the nurse would suggest that the doctor was patient-centered and that the nurse was task-centered and concerned only with lists of equipment and tasks. The oral communication processes were not reflected in the written data.

When questioned, nurses readily talked about their clinical nursing knowledge, their clinical dilemmas, the values that were being made explicit in their work and the ways in which their culture and knowledge had been constructed. However, during these discussions nurses often presented me with unexamined reasoning, myths, and accounts of unexamined nursing actions. What was significant was that the nurses themselves did not engage in writing about their practice, despite my encouragement, confining instead their written communications to lists or point form notes to jog their memories (aid memories). Although each nurse was particularly articulate, they demonstrated the fear, shared by many people in the general community, of the perceived authority and permanency of the written word and its openness to public scrutiny and contestation. The oral basis underlying nursing culture

and their socialization as women with oral skills had not prepared them to engage in extensive and expressive written data
about their nursing practice as a basis for critique.

Visibility: Oral Communication in Clinical Practice

In the process of my research I followed particular nurses
around for their entire shift. These nurses varied in their experience and, therefore, in their role within the nursing hierarchy. An examination of notes made during these shifts shows
that the nurses received almost all of their information orally
and that they presented most of their information in the same
way. On an average nine-hour shift some nurses would spend
less than ten minutes reading information and about the same
time writing. This time span for reading would be made up of a
number of brief scans of the charts or notes. The writing time
generally consisted of recording data such as blood pressure
readings on charts and in the brief time allocated to writing up
the notes, often consisting of no more than three sentences.
During the remainder of the shift the nurses would be generally speaking to someone, either staff, patient, or relative, most
of their working time.

This oral communication is an essential part of the nursing role. Nurses are in a work situation that requires them to
deal with a wide variety of staff with specific needs and
demands, as well as with their colleagues, patients, and visitors. During one observation session I counted five nurses,
thirty-two other staff and students, three relatives, and twenty-
one patients on one ward. These five nurses had to negotiate
their work within a situation that was stressful, crowded, and
requiring constant interaction. To achieve their nursing goals
within the wider scope of the various needs of the patients,
their visitors, and the varied professionals present, meant that
the nurses needed to ask, reassure, explain, direct, confer, and
delegate. In other words they needed to keep the communication flowing by talking and listening. Not only is oral communication an essential part of the nursing role, but it is also an
essential part of the structures and routines that surround
clinical nurses. The shift begins with an oral handover. The
practices for the handovers differed on different wards but
essentially the same process occurs. The nurses on the new
shift are given an overview of the patients on the ward, and

then after being allocated their patient(s) they are given a more comprehensive review often at the bedside and by the nurse who is presently looking after the patient. During the day shift this oral handover is supported as nurses from the new shift work alongside the nurses from the present shift for two hours. This double shift time enables the staff to take meal breaks and to attend meetings but there is still a considerable amount of time in which the two nurses can confer about the patient's condition, identify any special needs, or demonstrate any distinctive features of technical interventions or nursing skills.

The oral tradition is intrinsic to nursing culture and is recreated daily in the formal and informal rituals in which nurses engage. These rituals of the oral bedside discussion, the oral handover, the oral reporting to other staff, the constant oral interaction with patients, relatives, and colleagues, combine to perpetuate an oral tradition as the basis of nursing culture. Perry (1986) suggests that the female and oral tradition of nursing—as opposed to the male, medical model of research, recordkeeping and constant documentation—is tied to a belief that nurses are "born, not made." This view is historically based and represents the blurring between professional nursing care and some of its activities, which can be paralleled in the roles of parents and other lay careers. It developed from an assumption that nurses were born with an instinctive knowledge of caring. This assumption reached its logical conclusion in the suggestion that as people were "born nurses," they will instinctively have access to the kind of knowledge that that is necessary for nursing and, therefore, not need to engage in documentation about nursing practice. This attitude supports the notion that all nurses "know" what to do and, therefore, do not need careful records of what has been done previously to guide them in their decision-making. For female nurses this "knowing" is presumed to arise from a "natural" role as career, nurturer, and homemaker.

For Perry (1985:63) the pressure of time and routines has also convinced many nurses of the irrelevance of recordkeeping—particularly in the face of institutional structures that support this view with unrealistic staffing levels, physical layout of the wards, management rules, and unsympathetic rosters. These structures are based on "a concern for cost-effectiveness and quantifiable goals." She claims that it is in the interests of the dominant groups in the healthcare system to maintain the oral tradition as the "commonsense" way for nurses to function. My observations would support this view and suggest that under the present structures nurse administrators and educators will continue to fight a losing battle in their attempts to encourage or coerce nurses into writing about nursing when all the structures support and value the continuation of an oral tradition. During observations I also became aware that much of the communication was not restricted to oral language. Nurses used gestures, facial expressions, and other nonverbal means to communicate knowledge. This was particularly apparent when they were talking to other nurses. The nonverbal mode of expression assumes common knowledge and understandings. In the following exchange from a handover at the bedside it is apparent that only someone who was present during this exchange, and who shared common meanings, would understand the nursing knowledge being imparted.

> I have had trouble with his leg...see...and that has affected this...it keeps kinking so I found that if I put this around here like this then if he moves involuntarily it doesn't kink. But you have to pull this here like this before you touch him so that he doesn't wrench it out.

This exchange makes no sense when reported without the nonverbal and contextual meanings contained in the brackets below.

> I have had trouble with his leg...see (she touches the patient on the right arm and the left leg spasms and moves sharply) and that has affected this...(points to tube draining a wound) so I found that if I put this around here like this (demonstrates the way that the tube has been stretched around the leg of the bed) then if he moves involuntarily it doesn't kink. But you have to pull this here like this (she demonstrates the way that the loop needs to be pulled) before you touch him so that he doesn't wrench it out.

Although this extended account enables the reader to be able to gain a generalized impression of the incident, it does not allow for any precise understandings of the contextually bound meanings that were being exchanged between the two nurses. To begin to unpick what occurred in this incident an outsider would need to ask a number of questions such as: What is the effect on the patient of this uncontrolled movement of the left leg? In what way is it causing problems for the nurse? What are the implications of this for the treatment of the patient? What is the standard practice for the placement of drainage tubes in this hospital/ward? How has the nurse solved her problem? What did she do that was different to the normal practice?

The nurse who was being shown the arrangement of the tube was not a regular nurse at the hospital. She did not ask any questions as a result of the demonstration and her nods and "hmms" suggested that she felt that she had acquired enough facts from her observation of the patient and the visual situation to be confident of coping with it. The exchange took less than a minute. However, if the first nurse had been required to document that information for another nurse, who was new to the hospital and the ward and with whom she would have no face to face contact, then her documentation would need to contain considerable detail. It would be essential to explain the problem, the usual practice, the way in which she had varied the practice and directions to detail the specific way in which the tube needed to be placed and pulled for the practice to be effective. When we consider that this was only a very small part of the overall handover, then it becomes apparent that clinical nurses are unlikely to attempt to provide written descriptions of the idiosyncratic and context-specific knowledge that is distinctive to, and necessary for, their individual patients. The oral tradition appears to meet the needs of the nurse for information about the patient and the state of the technology or of the significant others surrounding the patients, for demonstration, for the opportunity to ask questions for clarification, and for the boost to their confidence that results from seeing how another nurse has coped with the situation. These factors mean that the patient benefits in a variety of ways that would be impossible if nurses had to rely on the written word to convey their complex knowledge and decision-making process concerning their individual patients. The patient becomes "visible" to another nurse through the processes and practices of oral communication whereas they remain "invisible" to the nurse through the written record.

Why then are educators and nursing administrators anxious that nurses begin to detail their information about patients? Nurses have reported a number of reasons why nurses need to document their nursing practice. The first reason is related to legality. It is claimed that records need to be full and accurate to protect the interests of the staff in the case of malpractice suits or as evidence in court proceedings.

The second reason relates to the human frailty of the nurse. No person is infallible and is able to remember every important detail of each patient each day. Administrators suggest that if nurses document important information throughout the shift, then the information is not lost if for some reason the nurse is unable to give a handover or to recall all the details.

The third reason relates to the improvement of nursing practice. Charge nurses want nurses to detail the kind of information that is not contained in the charts and which relates specifically to the nursing of that patient. For example, when a charge nurse discussed the nursing notes with an experienced nurse, she pointed out that the information included was either useful for the doctor or the physiotherapist but did not give any information about the nursing care that had been provided to the patient. Under questioning, the nurse admitted that this patient had been able sit in the chair for five minutes on three occasions during the shift. As this was an unexpected improvement and one that had not been mentioned during handover, it was therefore possible that this treatment would not have continued in the next shift through lack of information about this aspect of the patient's development. Instead, the nurse reading the notes would have yet another record of the fact that the blood pressure was not stable, information that was already contained in the charts.

Clinical nursing care can be disguised by the mechanisms of recording that are designed to illuminate the situation and the care being provided. Abbreviations used by nurses in charting information can be interpreted widely leading to confusion. RIB, meaning "rest in bed," has a variety of meanings for different nurses about their clinical practice with patients. These meanings range from the bed rest of the comatose patient to the patient who is allowed to get up for toileting or showering and include the postoperative patient with complications who must not be gotten up under any circumstances.

The difficulty of these interpretations of the recorded care plan means that it is not uncommon to find the following kind of situation.

A nurse was asked to tell a patient who was not under her care that the patient's husband was on the phone at the nurse's station. She went into the patient's room and read the nursing notes and saw "R.I.B." recorded in the notes. She was not sure whether this meant that the patient was allowed to get up at all or not so she asked the patient:

RN: Are you allowed out of bed?

Patient: I don't know; no one has told me that.

RN: Have you been up for anything?

Patient: I got up before and went to the toilet.

RN: Was a nurse with you?

Patient: No, I didn't tell the nurse.

RN: Well, I am not sure if your doctor wants you walking about or not. Your husband is on the phone. If you are allowed up you can go and speak to him, but if you are supposed to stay in bed I can give him a message.

Patient: Well, I'll go.

The nurse in this incident had not been given the oral handover to enable her to understand the meaning behind the abbreviation "RIB" for "rest in bed." Her action in allowing the patient to make an uninformed decision was poor clinical practice because she did not check the meaning with another staff member, and it was possible that the patient may have had serious complications from walking around. However, this kind of clinical practice is not unusual in the situation of a busy surgical ward, understaffed through the staff mealtime break. The nurse in this observation was very busy and relied on her clinical experience of these kind of surgical patients and on the common sense of the patient. If the information had been accurately recorded the nurse would have had a better understanding of the particular care plan for this particular patient. Some nurses use terms such as "strict RIB" or "RIB with T.P."

(toilet privileges) to elaborate, but even these terms appeared to be interpreted differently by different nurses. Therefore, it is apparent that nurses write nursing notes and care plans in a form that assumes that they will be able to provide the meanings behind the information orally. This assumption shapes the written format as a record of memory jogs to support the oral communication rather than as a record of care and projected plan of care.

Nurse researchers and educators are concerned that the oral tradition in nursing has denied other members of the nursing profession access to the knowledge that is being created and transformed by isolated individuals and groups engaged in clinical practice. Important new insights and knowledge are generated within clinical practice but are lost to the profession as a whole and, at times, to the individual nurse involved through the lack of a process by which nurses can examine their own practice and create and share new knowledge with their colleagues.

> It is a luxury for nurses to be able to take time to sit and think about some issues. We are not really encouraged to think about things. You don't have the time to sit with other nurses and talk together about things that bother you, so many nurses turn off. It's hard because you are not encouraged to talk or write about nursing, so you don't know how to...there are so many little incidents that really get to you over time...like the commission on death and dying (Dying With Dignity). I had lots of examples in my head, but I didn't have the whole picture—not the full case study, so I didn't know how to put it together.(RN, ICU)

The consequences of structuring clinical nursing so that nurses are not encouraged to talk and write about their clinical practices as a normal part of their work, is found in the invisibility of the idiosyncrasies of the individual patients in the written records, the invisibility of creative clinical practices, the invisibility of the connoisseurship of clinical nurses, and the invisibility of the ethics that are informing and shaping clinical decision-making processes.

11

❦

She's Just a Born Nurse

The myth of the female who was born to nurse casts its shadow over modern nurses. As with all myths its power lies in the fact that it has become part of the heritage of our language and so has the power to persuade us that it may be true. Even though rational thinkers would repudiate this myth, there are enough highly skilled practictioners of nursing who appear to embody the concept of the "born nurse," to cause confusion. The relationships that society constructs between nursing, mothering, homemaking, and femininity have meant that the role of nursing has been culturally submerged into what women do within our culture. The development of an understanding of the distinctive role of the nurse is difficult.

Power/Knowledge and the Nursing Role

Nursing staff are required to provide patient care for twenty-four hours each day, generally organized around three shifts of nine hours providing an overlap between nurses. This provision of continuous care has meant that the nursing role has developed a focus of enhancing the "personhood of the patient/client in the context of health related activities" (Marles 1988:17). This claim cannot be made uniquely by nurses because it is also the focus and preserve of other health professionals. Therefore, the generalist nature of the nursing role and the fact that nurses are available to the patient and their families when other health professionals are off duty means that many nursing functions overlap with the work of other health professionals causing confusion and a general lack of appreciation of the complexity of the nursing role. Clinical nurses themselves find it difficult to describe their role and so often resort to descriptions of the basic tasks unique to nursing in relation to the bodies of their patients, thereby ignoring the role of the nurse as interpreter of the healing process to the patient and their family. This interpreting role is aimed at ensuring that the medical and technological interventions necessary for the provision of a life-enabling environment for the patient do not violate or diminish the personhood of the patient. The nurse interprets the medical/health environment to the patient and their family and the needs of the patient and family to other health professionals. The difficulty that nurses have explaining their evolving role has led to a devaluation of nursing by other health professionals and by nurses themselves. Role conflict has occurred between nurses and paramedics and between nurses and doctors. This role conflict has become more pronounced as nurses value their role as nurses and challenge the power/knowledge relations in the health field.

Nursing Role: Continuity of Care

The role of the nurse involves the provision and maintenance of a life-enabling environment for the patient, which can include the provision of care and comfort in the dying process. A key aspect of this provision is the continuity of basic physical care. Constant observation of the patient using all the senses is necessary to ensure quality care. According to Eve:

> The doctors play around with technology but a good nurse watches the patient. You don't need all those monitors to tell you if the patient is all right. You can tell by carefully observing your patient.

With an unconscious patient this constant observation is essential as a tool for the treatment and prevention of problems as is evident in my observations of the care provided by Ann to her unconscious patient during a fifteen-minute period.

> Ann has just returned from morning tea and so she checks over her patient. She describes his needs as general nursing care. She comments that his special needs at

the moment are the fact that he has a bad sore on his bottom which means that he can't stay on his back too long, and that his respiratory function is still intact, so Ann wants to try to wean him off the ventilator. She tells me that she doesn't know if the patient can hear her or not but she always works as if he can as "they say that hearing is the last thing to go when they are unconscious." She touches him and tells him that she is going to clean out his mouth. As she suctions out his mouth she continues to speak to him as if he was responding. She says:

Well...lets clean out your mouth. I am going to suction out this tube to make you feel better. I will just move your head over here to straighten out the tube and make you more comfortable...OK now, you have a clean mouth.

Then Ann checked the patient's eyes again telling me that she will need to keep a careful watch on them as it appears that he is getting conjunctivitis. Ann gives the patient an eye toilet.

Then she tests for stomach acid.

Next, she checks his position and decides to move him onto his side because of the pressure on the sore on his back.

She touches him again before she speaks. She says:

I am going to put you on your back now.

Ann prepares to turn the patient. I ask her if she will be able to turn him by herself. She explains that she can do it because the patient is a dead weight. He has a flaccid response indicative of brain damage. This means that he stays where she puts him rather than rolling back onto her. Ann then turns the patient in stages until she has him comfortable. Ann takes particular care with this patient's head as it is very floppy. She also has to negotiate the placement of his tubes so that they continue to function.

Ann is providing this patient with routine nursing care. Although much of the nurses' role involves following doctor's orders for the patient, Ann is making independent decisions on the provision of physical care for her patient. This care is carried out in a physical environment that is maintained for the patient by the nurse. The nurse needs to ensure that the patient has adequate air through natural ventilation or the use of a ventilator and to take responsibility for deciding when the patient needs assisted air intake or needs to be weaned off the ventilator. The provision of appropriate light and warmth depending on the specific needs of the individual patient is another aspect of the nursing role. Here the nurse is responsible for making the required changes at the appropriate time for the patient's optimum health and comfort. The nurse is responsible for the technological interventions and the supervision of drugs and food/drink intake. The nurse regulates noise and visitors, often a challenging role requiring sensitivity and diplomacy. The individuality of the optimum health environment is evident in further notes from Ann's work with the aforementioned patient.

The nurse gives the patient another mouth toilet and checks his eyes.

The wife asks:	Are his eyes moving?...they aren't are they?...Can you tell?
Ann:	The doctor can do tests to check eye movement.
Wife:	I don't know what to do for him.
Ann:	Does he like music?
Wife:	Yes, he loves it. He always has the radio on at home.
A:	What kind of music does he like?
W:	Classical.
A:	Do you have a headset that you could bring in? I don't know if or when he can hear, but they say that the hearing is always the last to go.
W:	That's a good idea. I could bring in some of his tapes.

A: We do have a radio in here, but it is usually up the other end and mostly the nurses put it onto the stations they like because they don't know what the patients like or if they can hear it anyway. We have a Greek patient up the end, and his wife bought him a walkman, and we play Greek tapes all day for him.

W: That's a good idea. Yes...yes, I can do that. I am sure that would help him to respond.

A: Well if you bring it, we will make sure that he can have it on...I don't need to do anything for him for a while so I will do my work at the desk, and you can have some time by yourself with him.

The wife leaves the unit to make a phone call about the walkman and I ask Ann how she decides what information she should give to relatives, how, and when. Ann talks to me about her nursing:

As you can see this patient is keeping me very busy today even though he is stable. When we are involved with patients who are unstable then the nursing care tasks get left until there is time but this patient needs lots of nursing care—eyes, mouth, skin, turning. Then it always takes longer with the relatives. It is not so bad when there is only one...and that lady today...well she is easy because she doesn't get in the way and she is calm.

It is different with each patient. Some relatives don't want to know much. Others ask questions and when you start to explain they get upset so you don't go on too much. It depends if I have had contact with them before and if they have been into ICU before. Some people are so freaked out by this place that it doesn't matter what you say because they won't take anything in. I try to answer questions and tell them things I think I would want to know if I was them.

With this lady...well I tell her a lot because I was with her when the doctor told her of her husband's grim situation so I know what she has been told and I can give her more

information when she asks. She is also used to ICU now
and she is ready to take in much more information than
when her husband first arrived.

In this case it is evident that the patient is totally dependent on Ann for his physical needs. Although he is unconscious, Ann continues to interpret the hospital world to him by
telling him what she is going to do and why. She also interprets the patient's current health situation, his needs, and
future expectations to his wife.

Nurturance/Knowledge and Clinical Judgement

Ann uses her clinical judgement to nurture the patient
and the relatives through the provision of physical nursing
care and supervision of the proscribed curative activities in the
context of interpersonal relationships and a role as interpreter.
Although Ann was caring for a very sick patient she was able
to concentrate on his specific care needs without too many
interruptions. This is often not the situation in this busy ICU
or on a busy ward. Clinical judgement generally has to be exercised in the midst of constant interruptions, potential and real
crises and on behalf of more than one person at a time. The
unpredictability of clinical practice means that nurses need to
develop clinical judgement under the stress of constantly
changing scenarios. The following extract from my notes concerns the unpredictable actions of a patient, Mr. B, within a
busy morning for Carol:

9:50 a.m.:   Carol began filling in the patient board.

Carol: Sometimes it is hard to decide what to put
               against some patients. The staffing allocation
               is done on the number of points but some of
               these categories don't take into account what
               we have to do for some patients who are con-
               fused. Ahh!! Speaking of the devil (at this
               point a patient wandered into view holding
               out his urine bag)...Now Mr. B, what are you
               doing here? Going for a walk?

Patient: Yes, yes (nods happily).

Carol: Alright, but perhaps it would be a good idea

> to walk in this direction so you don't get lost.
> We don't want to lose you do we? (Carol
> turned the patient around and pointed him
> back in the direction of the ward).

Carol continued to fill in the board. The phone rang, and
she was told that a doctor was organizing a transfer of a
patient from another ward. She rang the charge nurse of
that ward and asked for details about the patient. Then
she went back to the board and added the name of the
new patient and using the information she had been given
and some educated guesses she made decisions about the
kinds of nursing assistance this new patient was likely to
need. The phone rang, and Carol gave details about a
patient's progress to a relative. As she was speaking Mr. B
reappeared at the nursing station and put his urine bag
on top of her notes. Carol finished the phone conversation
and said to Mr B:

Now Mr. B, I really don't want your bag here. Now you
carry it and I will take you back to your bed.

At this point a nurse appeared and said:

Oh Mr B, I have been looking for you. Your cup of tea has
arrived. Lets go back to your room, and I will find a comfortable chair for you to sit in while I make your bed. We
might empty that bag, too, it looks a bit full.

The nurse propelled Mr. B in the direction of his room and
said to Carol:

RN: I am sorry about that. Mr. A had just knocked his
cup of tea all over him so I was busy fixing him up
and didn't see Mr. B get out of bed. He is so quick,
and you don't know where he will go next.

Carol returned to the patient board and told another RN
to head off any more interruptions as she had to finish
the tally in time to get it sent down. Mr B wandered into
sight again with his urine bag. He started off down the
corridor out of the ward so Carol called out to the RN
responsible to come and collect him. Carol said to me:

He won't get too far as the wards on this floor connect and
eventually he will arrive back here.

Mr B arrived back on the ward escorted by an RN from the adjacent ward: "Does he belong to you Carol?"

Carol: Yes, that's Mr. B. He is feeling very energetic this morning, aren't you Mr. B?

Carol then asked an SEN to take Mr B for a long walk around the circuit of the four adjourning wards.

Later Carol went back and relieved the RN on the drug round. The RN went back to her section but reappeared and told Carol that she had "lost Mr. B." Carol suggested that she send the SEN to look for him.

The SNO arrived to talk with Carol about the staffing arrangements. As they began discussion a consultant on a round with his resident wanted clarification from Carol on the current arrangements being made by the family for the patient's accommodation after discharge. Carol told him about the kind of nursing care the patient was requiring and suggested that it would be unwise to return the patient to her own home unit straight away. Carol suggested that special accommodation might need to be considered for a short time.

Carol was called to the phone and asked if she had lost a patient. Apparently Mr. B had been found wandering out the ground floor entrance holding his urine bag. Carol called the RN and told her to go down to the lobby and get him. The RN was worried at first but Carol and I laughed so much at the image of this patient walking out on the front street in his pyjamas with his urine bag held aloft that the RN relaxed and agreed it was funny. She sped off downstairs to retrieve Mr. B.

The pharmacist arrived and told Carol that everyone downstairs (the pharmacy department is in the foyer) was very amused at the sight of Mr. B wandering out. She reviewed the stocks in the pharmacy cupboard with him and made some requests.

The RN arrived back with Mr. B in tow. She was very embarrassed at losing a patient, but Carol reassured her that Mr. B was unpredictable and that the problem was that the ward did not have enough staff to watch over patients who went walkabout. She then discussed the possibility of moving patients around so that they could put Mr. B in a single room so that his door could be kept shut. As Mr. B was totally disoriented by this time the RN put him in his bed with the sides up and tied his urine bag firmly to the bed. Carol went to see him to ensure that he was not upset by the incident and was comfortable.

Carol was required to exercise her clinical judgement in a variety of ways to deal with the problem of Mr. B within the context of the busy ward where she was responsible for patient care and for the work of her nursing team. She was aware of Mr. B.'s disorientation and of his response to medication, which was making him restless. In the middle of a busy schedule she had to keep responding to the needs of Mr. B. and the staff involved with him. The other activities in which she was engaged were important and needed concentration and the exercise of her clinical judgement. Carol had to handle the interruptions and constantly reassess the changed situation in relation to Mr. B in the light of her connoisseurship, her perceptual abilities, which included clinical knowledge, experience, intuition, and judgement.

Nurses such as Ann and Carol develop knowledge and clinical judgements about their patients and their health needs within a broader understanding of clinical nursing knowledge and the psychosocial world of the patient and the hospital. Engagement in these nurturant activities, which arise from, and with, their clinical knowledge, moves the nurse beyond the caring/curing/interpreting role into situations where nurses recognizes the power relations at work, which effect the well-being of their patients. These power relations become evident when the needs and interests of the hospital administration, the nurse, the other staff members or the patient's relatives supercede the needs of the patient. Clinical nursing judgements do not occur in isolation but in a sociocultural setting, which has been constructed by both power/knowledge relations and nurturance/knowledge relations. The interplay between the elements of power/knowledge and nurturance/knowledge provides a creative dialectic, which constructs and constrains clinical nursing. The exploration of this dialectic requires an exploration of the potentiality of nurturance/knowledge within clinical nursing roles as well as the role conflicts which constrain and maintain power/knowledge. Eve explained how she understood the roles of nurses.

The nurse at the bedside is the patient caregiver. To be effective in this role the nurse needs to be able to make an assessment of all the patient details—history, drugs, reasons for admission to hospital and to that particular unit or ward, whether the specific problems are current or recurring, specific care needed, potential difficulties, ongoing outpatient care, patient education. They should be able to evaluate every system and unite them into an understanding of that individual's problems and necessary nursing care.

Clinical Nursing: Role and Accountability

In order for nurturant action to be enabling, transforming, and person-centered, it must also be accountable to those people within its focus. Eve describes the manner in which nurturant activities create and reconstruct clinical knowledge and in turn are challenged and informed by this changed knowledge.

I expect the nurse in charge to check the work of the nurse at the bedside, to be accountable and to make the nurse accountable for their work. Most nurses and associate charge nurses don't like that idea. They think that only the untrained nurses need supervision and that when a nurse has graduated from the course she should know what to do.

According to Eve, clinical practice needs to be informed by clinical knowledge, and nurses should be held accountable to patients, relatives, staff, and the community for nursing actions. During an exploration of what it means to provide supervision, Eve explained:

I want nurses to be teaching professionals, so I have told the senior nurses that when they are in charge they are responsible for all nursing care in the unit, so they need to check what is going on. Some of them have found this difficult because they were used to all the nurses having their own tasks in their own bays. They felt like they were interfering, but what I want is for them to help develop the nursing care.

In the process of observing Eve at work it became apparent that she regarded herself as a teaching professional who recognized that the development of quality nursing care was an ongoing process with reciprocal accountability for the development of clinical judgement.

10:35 a.m.	Eve then went to the another bay to check on a new ICU graduate. She checked the settings for assisted breathing and questioned the nurse:
Eve:	Did you set this or was it done by the doctor?
Nurse:	I did, but (the intern) checked it.
Eve:	How did you make your decision to set it this way?
Nurse:	This is the setting that the doctor had Mr H (another patient) on the other day. He was also having respiratory problems, so I set it the same.
Eve:	Do you understand what the settings are for and what they are supposed to do?

The nurse gave an explanation.

Eve:	You are partly right. Do you understand the long-term effects of this amount of assisted breathing?
Nurse:	Not really. I know that they will be intubated longer.
Eve:	That's right, and that can lead to problems later. I will go through each setting and explain what they do, why they are used, and how they affect each other.

Eve then explained in detail what each setting is used for.

Eve:	Now what do you think the settings should be now?
Nurse:	Should I reduce it to 6?
Eve:	No, that is still too high for this patient.

Eve then explained in more detail why a lower setting was desirable.

Nurse: But wouldn't it be safer to have it at a higher level post-op and then reduce later?

Eve: Let's revise what happens to the patient with assisted breathing.

Eve then went on to discuss the patient's physiology and its relationship to the technical intervention and supports provided in the unit. As she talked she used her hands to indicate the sites on the patient that were interacting with the technology and the kind of changes that the technology was producing in the patient.

You can see how this is contracting when I put pressure here. That is the effect that this tube has on this system.

A lot of patients have...

Many patients react this way...

Some patients have...

Eve continued to explain the reasons for particular choices of settings and to highlight the differences in approach for different kinds of patients. Eve sees her role as charge nurse as a nurturant role, which is supportive of staff members both personally and in the development of their clinical knowledge and skills, while holding herself accountable to them, and them accountable to her, and to their patients. The following account demonstrates this kind of accountability in action as Diane, an associate charge nurse in the same unit, recognizes her moral accountability to provide emotional support to a junior nurse who had a very unpleasant task to perform and who was experiencing physical isolation from the others in the unit.

Diane expressed concern to me that a junior nurse would be required to change a dressing on a large open chest wound after the patient had been on dialysis. She said that although the nurse was perfectly capable of doing the dressing alone, she was determined to be with her for moral support as the wound not only smelled bad but looked quite frightening as all the patient's inner parts were exposed. The nurse had been alone in the bay for much of the time with the curtains closed because of the need to maintain sterile conditions. Diane kept her eye on the bay all morning and when it was time for the nurse to do the dressing we scrubbed up and Diane went to work with her while I tagged along. Diane introduced me to the nurse and the patient and we all put on fresh gowns and masks. The nurses put on fresh gloves and removed the dressing exposing the gauze which covered a large opening in the chest wall. Then the packing was removed from the wound exposing the interior of the chest and all the organs. The stench was overpowering. Diane kept talking to the semi-conscious patient reassuring her and encouraging the nurse. With the interior chest wall open the nurse used tweezers to drag sterile dressings over the wound to clean it. Diane inspected the wound, and checking that I was coping with the sights and smells she sent me to get the ward clerk to page the specialist. When informed that he had left the hospital she had the resident on duty paged. When he arrived and scrubbed, she said, "I want you to look at this wound now and write it up so I can be sure that someone (meaning a doctor) has seen it today. I don't want it to be opened again later, it's not fair on anyone." The doctor got the notes and examined the wound. He then wrote up the notes, checking details with Diane and the nurse as he wrote.

Diane not only held herself accountable for the support of the junior nurse but was accountable to the patient. She recognized the distasteful nature of the procedure and the extreme discomfort being experienced by the patient and so took initiatives to spare the patient a repeat procedure by organizing the resident medical officer to examine and document the condition of the wound. She acted as interpreter of the nurse's needs for emotional and moral support and interpreter of the patient's needs for comfort and dignity to the doctor. Diane's nurturing care included me as she was accountable to the patient, for my presence in the setting, and to me by providing a necessary commentary on the procedure while checking that I was coping with the observation.

These examples occurred in the highly technological ICU unit and related to very specific nursing skills and knowledge, which required a mastery of patient physiology and the effects of various technical interventions on the patient. This technical knowledge and the ability to act appropriately and efficiently in the use of highly sophisticated and constantly changing technology is essential in a critical care nurse. Eve and Diane also demonstrated their interpretive capacities and their abilities to "connect" with the temporality of the patients. Eve used her extensive clinical experience of observing patients on ventilators to enable her to foreshadow the consequences, to the patient, of the legitimate but overly cautious ventilator settings of the graduate nurse. The graduate nurse and the intern were focusing on the specific needs of that particular patient, at that moment, in the light of their textbook knowledge of the patient's condition and ventilation procedures. By contrast Eve was considering the patient in the light of her knowledge of his personal medical and social history, current situation, and expected pattern of healing, and in the light of her experience of nursing hundreds of patients on ventilators. Eve was combining her technical "knowing that" with her practical know-how to provide a perceptual knowing that is temporal and context-specific, a concept which Polanyi (1962) describes as "connoisseurship." Connoisseurship recognizes the qualitative judgements involved in clinical knowledge, a perceptual, intuitive grasp of the whole situation, which can never be reduced to sets of rules to be technically applied in the situation.

Clinical Judgement and Transformative Action

In each of these exemplars of clinical knowledge in action the nurses moved beyond the role of interpreter to engage in transformative action. Eve valued her clinical knowledge more highly than the technical know-how of the graduate nurse and the intern. She put the interests of the patient first by allowing her connoisseurship to prompt action that was transformative for this patient by reducing his dependence on the ventilator and facilitating a faster, safer route to independence. Diane's connoisseurship and her empathy for the nurse and the patient prompted her to ignore potential problems from the medical specialist and to act in the interests of the patient.

The legacy of the legitimation of the technical basis of nursing culture with its emphasis on objective, value-free knowledge practiced in an objective context creates dilemmas for nurses who constantly experience the intersubjective nature of nursing. This technical view contends that nurses need to be able to take an objective view of the patient and the activities in which the nurse engages on behalf of the patient. The dilemmas emerge when nurses engage in emancipatory actions on behalf of their patient in a nursing culture committed to technical action. The hierarchy of knowledge within the hospital culture legitimates technical knowledge; although nurses challenge this technical culture by their clinical practices, they accord technical knowledge superiority and judge their own practices accordingly. Although Diane is considered a highly skilled clinical practitioner with expert technical knowledge, she claims that she is not a "good" ICU nurse because she is unable to maintain objectivity:

> It is always a conflict in my work. That's one of the reasons why I am not very well organized at work. I put off doing things because I can't maintain that objectivity that I need to be a really good intensive care nurse...of being able to do the task-oriented things you need to do when you are supposed to...I prioritize differently to the way I feel I should prioritize...How much sleep someone gets, how comfortable they are feeling emotionally, if they are awake enough to be involved in that sort of thing, and giving them a say in their own care...in a situation which is basically dehumanizing, to me those things are very important.

> I can remember nights when I did no physio on someone all night because they were feeling really "agro" and "anti" and didn't want to be touched, and I thought well that's your decision and I can explain to you the reasons why I should be doing those things but if you don't want that then that's your decision. I would be really sweating on the x-ray the next morning and thinking if she has developed her basal collapse again I will kill myself and then breathing a great sigh of relief when she hadn't. But these are things that a proper objective person would never do.

> A.S.:   I don't really believe that your definition of a proper objective nurse is really what you want to be.

> Diane: No, it's not what I want to be at all. I mean I realize there is a place for those people but it isn't me. I get involved...It is the main thing that keeps me in nursing—the relationships. Last Saturday when I was working with Sally, I spent all day

talking with her. I hardly did any obs. at all. Sally
can't speak properly so you have to lipread her.
That makes it a slow job communicating with her
at all. After sitting down with her I discovered that
she had been experiencing uncontrolled pain that
we (the nurses) had not recognized because we
had been too busy to take the time to sit down
and talk with her. When I discovered what her
problem was we were able to do something about
it. She told me that she had been reluctant to go
home because she was afraid of dying at home
without adequate pain control. Sally is a very
intelligent woman, she knows what is happening
to her, and she knows what she needs.

This patient had experienced excellent technical care supported by nursing observations and physical care, however,
even her medical needs were not being met because the routines of the ward militated against placing a priority on communication. The technical culture of the ward denied Sally the
technical intervention she desperately needed in the form of
pain control. A subsequent discussion with Sally disclosed the
fact that prior to Diane's clinical care, she had been planning
suicide to escape from her pain. The instigation of appropriate
pain control by Diane meant that Sally was able to go home
comfortably to enjoy family life before she died. Diane recognized that in this instance communicating with the patient was
more important than engaging in a multiplicity of technical
tasks. She trusted her clinical judgement to abandon these
tasks in favor of communication because she felt confident
that she would recognize any changes in the patient's condition if she was sitting with her all day. She would not need to
rely on the information afforded by the different measuring
and monitoring devices because her own perceptions were able
to recognize subtle physiological changes. Diane's clinical
judgement in this instance transformed Sally's life by liberating her from severe pain and the fear of a painful death.

Clinical Nursing: Role Relations

An analysis of the clinical nursing role needs to be conducted in the context of the roles of other health professionals.

Traditionally nurses have understood and evaluated their role in relation to the medical role. However, recent nursing scholarship has worked at providing conceptual models that describe the nursing role as a separate entity with a different focus to the medical role. These nursing frameworks focus on the whole person in contrast to the medical focus on the treatable part. In this way some nurses have attempted to describe nursing as a "science of caring" (Dunlop 1986) and medicine as a science of curing. Despite the obvious medical focus on cure, nurses can not claim a monopoly on caring activities. Many doctors provide their patients with care and cure, and many nurses are just as active in providing curative procedures as in caring activities. The difference in roles can be described more effectively in terms of the continuity of care provided by nurses involved in the curative process.

Role relations between doctors and nurses vary considerably between individuals, wards, and hospitals. Senior nurses and specialist nurses generally have different relationships with doctors than new graduates or experienced generalist nurses. These role relations are sometimes confused when nurses are forced to act in a more senior role on particular shifts. This role confusion was more apparent on the ward where as Brewer (1986) found, degrees of decision-making power, responsibility, and accountability varied for any particular nurse depending on the shift in which the nurse was working. There are always more senior nurses on the day shift, less on the evening shift, and often only one on the night shift. This means that an RN might be in charge of a night shift and yet could find that on a day shift there were three others above them in the hierarchy. This leads to some role confusion for the nurse, patient, and the doctor.

Doctor: Nurse can you come here and fix this dressing please.

RN who is acting in charge on this shift:
            I'll look for the nurse who's working in this room.

Doctor: But aren't you the nurse who was here yesterday morning and did the dressing for me?

RN: Yes but this evening I am in charge, and I have to see the nursing supervisor now about patient allocations. (RN, medical ward)

Doctor/Nurse Relations

The Marles report (1988) found that both nurses and doctors described a general deterioration in relationships between the two groups although their understandings of the reasons for the deterioration differed. Much of the conflict appears to emerge from differing nursing role expectations. In the past nurses have often acted as handmaidens for medical staff, and the Marles report contains evidence from medical groups judging modern nurses against this standard of service to the doctor, before service to the patient. Nurses who are able to respect themselves as equals with the medical staff still find it difficult to act in ways that are emancipatory because of their traditions, because of their embodiment in habits which they respond to on an unconscious level, and because of the behavior of the medical staff. In the following example, Diane typifies the actions of nurses who are changing the ground rules in the doctor/nurse game.

A new resident on the ward asked Diane to help him with a procedure.

Diane (to me):   He wanted to know how to do a procedure. It is a medical procedure, and he should have been taught it by a senior anaesthetist, but those men leave it to the senior nurses to show their juniors. We show them how, but we don't do the procedures. We are not allowed. It is a medical procedure.

Dr: I need some ice.

Diane: You will need to get a bucket to put the ice in. Do you know where they are kept?

Dr: No. (gesturing helplessly).

Diane: The buckets are kept in the storeroom over there. (Diane went on to explain where the buckets could be found and then where he could get the ice)

The resident wandered off but was soon back.

Dr: I can't find the buckets.

Diane: They are under the bottom shelf.

Diane continued to care for her patient, and the resident arrived back with the bucket and no ice. So Diane again explained where the ice was kept. The resident wandered off with his bucket.

A.S.:   Did that doctor expect you to get the ice for him?

Diane: I wouldn't. It's for a medical procedure. He does the procedure, and he should know where to get the things that he needs...Actually that resident is pretty good. He doesn't expect you to do everything for him. Some doctors would stand by and expect you to do the fetch and carry tasks. I used to do them for the doctors but now I don't.

A.S.:   I think you handled it well. He looked so helpless that I could feel the temptation to go and do it for him rather than go on and on explaining.

Diane: Yes, it is important not to get sucked into mothering the interns and residents.

The resident came back without the ice one more time, and Diane patiently explained again. He finally arrived back with ice in the bucket. (Diane, ICU)

These changing relationships are developing as nurses are beginning to recognize the value of their clinical knowledge gained through continuous care relationships with their patients. However, this component of continuous care leaves them tied to the bedside and separates them from the opportunities for impromptu professional development through discussions with other health professionals.

11:45 a.m. Thursday. We went into the staff room for a morning tea break as Diane had been too busy to take a break earlier with other staff. We found the Unit director and two anaesthetists discussing new ideas and techniques. This had developed naturally from the ward round held at 9 a.m. this morning. Although Diane as associate charge nurse had been present at the ward round she had been continually interrupted and constantly required to return to the unit to assist her nursing staff. As we left,

Diane said: "Wouldn't it be good to be paid to sit and talk about nursing half the day."

A little later Diane was informed that as a result of that discussion between the doctors, a dying patient was to be given a new treatment. This patient was severely brain damaged as a result of a suicide attempt to escape from the constant pain of an incurable disease. The nurses involved were unhappy and clustered together to discuss the situation. They expressed their concern that the doctors did not expect the patient to live but wanted to try out the new technique. Nurses commented that they were just "using" the patient for their own experiments. Diane told me that she was unhappy about the decision, which would involve time and resources for a patient that everyone was sure would die anyway. She suggested that it may prolong the patient's life unnecessarily.

Diane went to the doctor in charge and asked if the proposed treatment was necessary. The doctor responded that it could have a slight chance of success, and it was their role to preserve the patient's life if they could. (Diane, ICU)

Although Diane had been present at the ward round discussion on this particular patient, she had not been able to participate in the informal discussion which occurred after the official round had finished. It was during this time that the doctors rescinded their original orders to maintain the patient in comfort without further interventions, deciding instead to instigate a new technique. Diane did not hear about the changed treatment plan until the doctors had already begun to implement it. The nurses were not considered equal team members holding particular clinical knowledge necessary to the decision-making process. In this case the nurses working with the patient had particular experience with the family and the patient which informed their clinical judgements of the appropriate care for this patient. The doctors' ethical considerations were directed to the saving of life whereas the nurses' ethical considerations were focused on the potentialities in the quality of life for the patient and his family. The inequalities structured in the role relationships between the medical staff and the nursing staff meant that these ethical dilemmas were not debated. These structured inequalities between nursing and medical staff are further complicated by the inequities experienced by women in the workplace. According to Carol:

> One of the big problems for nursing is that most nurses are women, and so they have problems in being accepted as an equal with other staff. They don't help this because they see themselves as inferior to the doctors and other paramedics. Even with the increase in male nurses, it doesn't help the women much because the male nurses float to the top and the female nurses let it happen. They need their consciousness raised. They accept a submissive role. But still you have to be careful with male doctors not to overreact if you have a problem and you want to get something done. You have to be assertive just to be noticed, and then they say, "oh what's got into you today." It becomes your fault; you have the problem and they can forget about you. It's a no-win situation. It is hard for young female nurses especially when they are new to the hospital. When you are older and have been in the hospital for a long time, then you become more comfortable with yourself. However, there are always times when you have to assert yourself as a professional person because you are a woman. Men assume that they will be in charge, whereas women need to be given permission to be in charge as men take control without assessing individual ability.

> The men also assume that what they do is alright because they are doctors. I saw two medical staff stand at the end of a patient's bed and, ignoring the patient and his male visitor, they discussed the patient's problem of impotence. How rude and unprofessional! I was so mad, I called them out and roared them up. But that's hard to do, and even if those doctors remember there will be another one the next day who will do the same kind of thing.

> This kind of arrogance by many male doctors and the submissive attitude of most female nurses means that the nurses will go to any lengths so that they won't be shown up in front of a doctor. Once when I was leaving to go home a nurse asked me to come back and see a patient. When I told her to get the resident to see the patient and ask for a referral, she said that she couldn't "because he might make me feel small."

In making these comments Carol is generalizing about female nurses and male doctors. However, her comments are consistent with my observations of doctor/nurse relations during the research and with the experiences recounted by many other nurses. Carol discussed the changes in relationships experienced by nurses with interns, the older son in the family symbolism, and the changes when they inherit the mantle and become doctors.

When interns start on the wards, they need the help of the charge nurses so they are often OK to you, but later when they become experienced doctors, they ignore you.

Nurses accept a lot of this because they don't have enough self-esteem. They take unnecessary crap from doctors. They don't believe that they have professional knowledge and skills. Many of them need to grow up and realize that not everyone will like them. It is a big world out there. While they try to be liked by everyone, they will not be able to develop professionally. They need to be more aware of issues in nursing and not just their personal emotions. They need to be able to stand up for themselves and not be held responsible for medical decisions that are wrong because they are afraid of the doctors or because they want them to like them.

Many nurses play the doctor/nurse game. I think that it is more subtle now than when we used to stand up when a doctor entered a room and let them walk in front of us through doors and things like that. Nurses allow the doctors to treat them as inferior, but the doctors don't treat the paramedics in that way. They are seen to be equals. Nurses are still expected to go and find things for medical staff as if their own work was not as important. The doctors would never ask a paramedic to go and get something for them. Often the doctors don't bother doing their work properly because they know that a nurse will come along and finish it for them. If a doctor is asked to write up orders they will often start writing them on a blank chart. If you query the fact that they haven't put a patient label on the chart first they will say that they don't know where they are or that they thought that you would do it because they are in a hurry.

We need to state and restate that we are here for the patients and not for the doctors. When you are discussing patients with the doctors, it is often difficult for nurses to get the message across that they are interested in the patient's welfare and not the doctor's feelings or problems.

We have to change the (attitudes and actions of the) medical staff. You can tell that there is a gender problem because the female consultants don't have the same problems working with the nursing staff. They treat us more as equals. They will ask for your opinion or leave you to take responsibility for things. The sexual thing isn't there as you can't flirt with a female doctor.

Carol has astutely highlighted a number of issues in the gender role relationships, which are characterized in the relationships between doctors and nurses. She recognizes that the consequences for female nurses of being treated as less than equal has led many nurses to accept and support these inequities based on class and gender relations. Many nurses have developed tactics for survival, such as avoidance of interactions with medical staff, which perpetuate the problem. Other responses are typified by the kind of emotional immaturity that Carol highlights when she discusses the way in which many nurses want to be liked by everyone to the detriment of professional development and the pursuit of nursing issues. Doctors also indulge in this emotional immaturity and continue to expect that they will be the focus of the nurse's world with their needs preceding the needs of the patient. Carol suggests that this was fostered by senior nurses in the past who insisted that doctors be given special privileges, status, and support, but that nurses still contribute to their own oppression by participating in new, more subtle doctor/nurse games. This failure of the majority of nurses to challenge the status role claimed by the doctors means that when the minority try to act in ways that are assertive, their actions are characterized as demonstrating that there is something wrong with them, that it is the nurse who has a problem. According to Carol, doctors do not adopt the same role when working with paramedics as they do with nurses. Carol's experiences with female doctors has led her to the conclusion that gender roles are instrumental in medical hegemony. She identifies the effects of this hegemony in the assumption made by males that they will be in charge and the reluctance of women to challenge this situation without being given specific permission.

The consequences of these structured inequities were not only apparent in the role relations between the medical and nursing staff on the wards but extended to the decision-making processes in the hospital as Bev described:

> ...another thing that bugs me is that we (nurses) are told that we are all a team with the doctors and the physios and admin, but when it comes to making important decisions that affect us we are never consulted. An example is the situation that is happening now. The hospital administration and the senior medical staff have entered into an agreement with another hospital to do a particular operation for them. We, the senior nurses who have to do the work, weren't asked, the charge nurse wasn't asked, or even nursing admin. Its money really. The hospital gets $40,000 for each of these operations—not our unit, not us, but the hospital. That's how they make decisions that affect us. They just ignore us.

Administrative and Clinical Nursing Role Relations

The powerlessness resulting from unequal role relationships, which were often disguised by the appearance of token authority, were commented on frequently.

> Eve: The charge nurse has no real power. Admin checks up on all that we do. All the nursing supervisors do is check up on us, and then administration check up on them. For example, the rosters. I do them, and I know my staff. I know what they are capable of, what level they are at, what their personal and social situations are. It takes me ages to work out a roster, and then the supervisor comes along and has to check everything. She goes through them all, and then they go down to nursing admin who go through them all again...Sometimes I wonder why I need to waste time checking my work if it is going to be double-checked by admin. You can be less responsible when you don't have full responsibility for your work. They talk about devolution of power to the

areas, but they structure things so that we don't have any real power. We can make some limited decisions about how to spend some money on the unit, but we don't receive separate budgets, and we can't see where the money is or where it has come from. We can't be responsible for good management because we don't have the knowledge about how the budgets are constructed to enable us to make responsible decisions...I want to participate in the development of the future of nursing, but it is difficult when all your suggestions are ignored. The admin have control over the future of nursing in this hospital, and many of them haven't nursed a patient in years.

Eve's comments reflect the consequences to nursing of hierarchical power structures which rob nurses of the need to become responsible and accountable for their work. These structures support inequalities in role relationships and contribute to stereotyped responses between nursing administrators and clinical nurses. The comment that nursing administrators haven't engaged in recent clinical nursing practice is a common complaint from clinical nurses disenchanted with decisions that affect them but into which they have had no input. In turn nursing administrators point to mistakes and inadequacies in documentation to justify their need for supervisory processes.

Carol suggests that these hierarchical role problems are exacerbated by lack of clarity of role expectations:

We fall between two stools now. In the past the hierarchy was so clearly defined that it was easier to know what your role meant because you knew what was expected of you. It wasn't good, but it was easier. We haven't achieved the ultimate. I think that nurses need consciousness-raising groups to help us develop our understanding of our role.

Eve has a reputation throughout the nursing staff as a nurse who was very clear about the difference between medical and nursing roles. This clarity enabled her to aid patients, their families, and the medical staff. She has a commitment to her role as a nurse and to the distinctly different role of the medical staff, which enables her to challenge role inequities and at the same time be careful not to usurp the medical role inappropriately:

12:30 p.m. A group of relatives came to visit a male patient who was dying. They wanted to speak with the doctor, but as he was unavailable Eve spent time with them. Although she gave them as much information as she could, she also differentiated between what she knew about and what they would need to refer to the doctor. She then phoned the doctor's rooms and organized a time for the relatives to speak with him.

Hegemony and Accountability

According to Eve, many nurses perpetuate the status quo because they are not prepared to be held accountable for their actions and decisions. They resist examining their nursing role and developing it because this would not only involve individual action but would necessitate an examination of the culture of the unit and the manner in which the culture is re-created and maintained. Eve suggests that the nursing culture is changing, and in future nurses will need to develop their understanding of their role, their clinical knowledge, and their accountability.

Eve: I am interested in the kind of changes that will occur in nurses when they are expected to take responsibility for nursing the patients rather than acting as collectors of data for doctors. A lot don't want to change. They like the situation as it is because they don't really want to be held responsible for their nursing decisions and the care that they provide.

In reality most nurses are task-oriented rather than patient-oriented. This is really hard to change. It is like changing the culture of the whole unit. The nurses think that being a good nurse is completing a number of set tasks. This has been ingrained in them, and it is really hard to change. We have only a few excellent nurses who are thinking all the time about why things are happening. I expect all nurses to know all about their patient and be able to rationalize why the patient needs anything.

Even though some nurses are unable to do more than think in terms of tasks and systematic assessment, I think that they give holistic care because of their role at the bedside all day and because their tasks and assessments cover all aspects of the patient. Doctors only focus on the medical problem under treatment at the moment.

ICU nurses are much more experienced than the medical personnel working in ICU. The nurses often work in the unit for years and see the same kinds of cases over and over. The doctors come and go for only a short time so they may only see one or two cases of a particular kind before they move on. A study done on critical care asked doctors, paramedics, and nurses to predict the prognosis of patients in critical care units. The nurses were much more reliable at determining the prognosis of the patient than either of the other two groups.

The nurses are also much more familiar with the technology and its effects through constant use and experience. The doctors may understand what the technology can do and know how to use the data from textbooks, but their inexperience with the actual technology and its effects on patients means that their decisions may not be as appropriate to the particular situation. They tend to work from the technical data and not from the patient.

Eve is able to affirm the clinical knowledge of the nurses in her unit in relation to their ability to provide patient care and in the interface with the technology. She differentiates between the role of the practical knowledge held by the nurse and the technical knowledge held by the doctor. She also expects that the nurses should have the technical knowledge necessary to assess the patient and the technology and to act appropriately. Eve is able to recognize that nurses are limiting patient care when they are not prepared to think about it and to be held responsible for their clinical judgements and actions. She is identifying a need for nurses to engage in a process of enlightenment in order to engage in actions that are transformative, to develop emancipatory knowledge.

Power/Knowledge and the Gendered Body

Discussions of the relationships between power and knowledge in nursing action need to take account of the people who are engaging in these actions. Nurses are not disembodied subjects without history or culture. Nursing is a discipline that can involve the bodies of nurses in intimate relationships with the bodies of their patients or clients. The bodies of both nurses and patients are gendered bodies—bodies whose understandings and desires have been shaped and limited by the social construction of gender.

The Gendering of a Nurse

Nursing as a discipline dominated by females and subjugated to the the male-dominated medical profession, powerfully demonstrates gender relations. These gender relations are integral to an understanding of the actions of nurses because they are historically and culturally formed. This socially constructed gendering process begins long before women and men become nurses as is evident from the discussion between the following three nurses who are in their late twenties to early thirties:

Meg: My earliest memories of a connection with nursing come from when I was five and my seven-year-old brother went to hospital with a broken leg. He decided he wanted to be a doctor, and so I announced that I wanted to be one, too. My mother laughed and said: "No Michael can be a doctor, and you can be his nurse." My mother was talking about this again the other day, and she said, "It's so funny, you were so determined to be a doctor and we used to say "No, you will be a nurse." I knew even then, you are a born nurse." (groans from the group) Now, because I am a nurse she thinks that she knew best, but I wonder what would have happened if they hadn't started telling me that was what I would be?

Sandi: I know what you mean. I grew up in a medical family; my grandfather and father are doctors, but from when I was little everyone always talked about how I would be a nurse. I am an only child, and my father's friends used to make comments about how it was a pity he didn't have a son to follow in the family medical tradition but no one even considered that I could—including me. Most of my earliest play memories are being dressed in a nurse's uniform, looking after my dolls and pets. My photo albumn has a number of photos of me in nurse's uniform, so I guess I am what is called a self-fulfilling prophecy.

Meg: Yes!. My brother had a doctor's set, and I had a nurse's set. Even then he used to tell me what to do, I just followed on. Mind you now, he works as a retail salesman.

Meg and Sandi demonstrate the early socialization, which provided them with a gendered construction of what it meant to be female and tied that female construction to the occupation of nursing. They were not only denied the opportunity to imagine themselves in the role of a doctor, but the clothes they wore and the play activities they pursued were structured by their parents to reinforce the messages of nursing as an appropriate occupation for women. Of interest is the fact that although Meg's mother actively colluded in the construction of Meg's image of herself as woman in a woman's occupation, her own gendered socialization was so strong that she was unable to recognize the effect of her role in this process and could make the preposterous claim that Meg was a born nurse.

Meg and Sandi's experiences demonstrate very obvious forms of gendering, which are not shared by all women who enter nursing now, although there are many young nursing students who have similar stories. Changes in societal attitudes towards roles have opened up many other occupations to women, but have made little inroads on the establishment of nursing as a socially desirable occupation for men.

Phillip's experience of gendering was as sterotypical as Meg's and Sandi's but emerged from a different socially constructed and defined gender orientation. These differing gendering experiences demonstrated what Lipman-Blumen (1984:104) describes as latent socialization "the process whereby individuals are socialized indirectly to those roles the society does not expect them to perform on a regular basis." The families of both Meg and Sandi gave them specific messages, which demonstrated to them not only that nursing was an appropriate gender role but that medicine was not. Phillip also experienced this process of latent socialization, but whereas the two women acquiesed to their gendered destiny, Phillip provides an example of someone who challenged the gendering of occupational roles.

Phillip: My experience was very different. My parents wanted me to follow my father in the family business. I did economics and maths for higher school certificate and hated it. I began work in a bank and lasted less than six months. Then I did about six other jobs in two years. Finally I went to a career guidance counselor and did all the tests. Nursing was something that came up, and I immediately felt interested. My father was furious and demanded to know if I was gay. I told him that I wasn't, but he said well that's what everyone will think about you anyway.

The comment by Phillip's father concerning his sexual orientation demonstrates the relationship between the body and the culture of nursing. Female children are prepared for nurturant activites by initiation through play activities and rituals of dress, which imitate functions and social roles that are seen as socially desirable for females. Males who demonstrate an interest in what society ordains as essentially female nurturant roles are often labeled as deviant by the dominant culture, whether this label is appropriate or not.

Males and females in nursing report different experiences of treatment. Phillip reported that he was given experience "in charge" of the shift on the ward earlier than the female colleagues who were his contemporaries. Ruth, who works with Phillip, reported that she was more often given "housework" type nursing tasks than Phillip, whom she felt was more likely to be given administrative experience. She claimed that Phillip had more general independence on the ward, a claim supported by Phillip and other male nurses.

The gendering of the female body in nursing includes guidelines and rituals relating to clothing, hair styles, "ladylike" movement, conversational structuring, and body shape. These culturally legitimated bodily rituals reveal the body as a gendered text of culture (Bordo 1989), which is reflected in the stereotypes of media culture. These rituals reveal the myths of nursing, which transcribe a culture of docility on the bodies of nurses. The structuring of this docility is evident in Marie's comments:

This nursing uniform drives me mad because it restricts free movement. I wish we could wear trousers like the male nurses or female doctors. Our work involves an awful lot of moving around in all directions. I seem to be always lifting, carrying, repositioning patients, bathing, reaching for things and all the time we are supposed to look neat, tidy, and ladylike. It's crazy. It makes you more conscious of your self all the time because you have to pull down your skirt or tidy your hair. The guys just do their work without this image problem.

Bordo (1989: 14) argues that the contemporary obsession with appearance, which:

still affects women far more powerfully than men, even in our narcissistic and visually oriented culture, may function as a "backlash" phenomenon, reasserting existing gender configurations *against* any attempts to shift or transform power-realtions.

Bordo is highlighting the body as a text of femininity which contains not only symbolic meaning but *political* meaning. Through this symbolic and political meaning women's bodies can be shaped, limited, and controlled. Jane is a large woman who finds her image creates problems as a nurse.

I am a big woman. All the women in my family are, but we are also all active and healthy. However, there is this image that nurses are supposed to portray. I mean healthy nurses are supposed to be thin, and I feel myself constantly on the defensive because I'm not...We were talking about oppression before; well I feel oppressed as a woman in a man's world, oppressed as a nurse in this hospital and oppressed as a big woman.

I know it affects my work. The consultant on our ward is a big man, but it's OK for him to be big. He's a man and a medical specialist!

I think I am less assertive than I would like to be because I'm aware of my size.

The text of culture written on the bodies of Australian women has a story line that celebrates the slim, active woman who maintains the image of both health and femininity according to our cultural standards. Media and popular culture portray the nurse as either a young, slim, attractive woman or a tough, old disciplinarian, physically and socially unattractive. When faced with the meanings in these stereotypes nurses make choices, either consciously or unconsciously, to fulfill the attractive image. For those whose physical inheritance makes the task of conformity difficult, there is the task of attempting to conform, and for those who fit the image, the task becomes to maintain it.

The Gendered Body of the Patient

Changes in equal opportunity legislation restrict the official processes of gender discriminiation in the workplace, but the impact of the gendered body in nursing is still apparent in the attitudes of nurses and the the general community. Social attitudes to intimate contact with bodies is also constructed along gender lines as became apparent in a discussion I had with Phillip:

Phillip: When I went to wash Mrs G she was upset and asked to have a "nurse" wash her. When I explained that I was her nurse, she told me that she wasn't having a strange man touch her.

A.S.: Have you experienced this before?

P: Yes, but last time it was a man complaining that he wasn't having himself washed by another man. It's ironic isn't it—you can't win with either sex.

A.S.: It interests me because there is no consistency in this approach. As a woman I prefer to be cared for by female nurses, but I also choose to have a female doctor.

P: Yes you're right about the inconsistency. Mrs. G has a male doctor whom she raves about and who handles her more intimately in his internal examination than I would have done giving her a wash. She also forgets that her male surgeon has had very intimate contact with her when she was on the operating table.

A.S.: That's true, but she was not awake and looking him

in the eye as she would have been doing with you. Why do you think that the male patient you mentioned didn't want you to wash him?

P: I guess he thought I might make sexual advances because perhaps, like my father, he thinks all male nurses are gay.

A. S.: He would need to have a female doctor, to be consistent, if he thought that male health workers might make sexual advances to him or embarass him, but I presume he has a male doctor.

P: Yes, he does, and because he has trouble with his prostrate he has had examinations of his genitals by his doctor. Its funny now when I think about it because he wanted to have me shave his face...but he let her (female RN) shave his genital area.

Culture has essentially delegated the role of nursing to women and the effect of this is evident when members of the community need to be hospitalized and to take on the role of patient. Activities that are deemed to belong to the domain of nursing have been designated "women's work." Invasions of bodies through surgery and internal examinations are considered to be appropriate for medical practitioners and so are acceptable, whereas washing has been defined as an appropriate female role causing some concern to patients when this unacknowledged cultural assumption is violated. The male patient differentiated between public areas ("because he wanted me to shave his face") and private areas ("he let her shave his genital area") in a way that reflects the gendering of roles relating to different parts of his body and the meanings that they hold for him.

An early part of nursing socialization relates to ways nurses learn to deal with this intimacy with the bodies of strangers. Nurses learn to cope by objectifying the parts of the body with which they are dealing in order to protect themselves and their patients. The use of technical language aids this process of distanciation. An effect of this process is to turn the patient from a subject into an object of nursing care—the asthma patient in bed four.

This socialization of nurses is interesting when an examination is made of the distinction made by patients between the gaze of the doctor and the gaze of the nurse. The actions and reactions of these patients would suggest that the gaze of the doctor is classed as the observation and investigation of the objective scientist, whereas the gaze of the nurse is assumed to be the subjective gaze of person-to-person intimacy. This attribution of intersubjective relationship between patient and nurse places the relationship more in the private sphere than the public sphere. In this way both male and female patients may demonstrate the structuring of gender by expressing a preference to have nursing care provided by females, thereby reflecting social attitudes towards nurturant activities and the presumption that these activities are best carried out by women.

12

❦

Yes, But You'll Never Change That!

A common complaint of nurses is that they are powerless to change anything. The phrase "yes, but" is a common part of the language of many nuses who have experienced their own powerlessness and have lost hope and enthusiasm for the struggle to effect change.

Hegemony in Clinical Practice

Hegemony was daily recreated and maintained by nurses and administrators by the nurses in the study. The mechanics of hegemony was particularly apparent in areas where nurses objected to the bureaucratic processes that had been instigated to deal with nursing issues, but yet they continued to act in ways which supported those processes. According to Diane:

> Nurses hate putting anything in writing...like nursing documentation. They hate doing it. They just hate putting it on paper. They hate words. They hate pens...I don't know why that is, whether that has been part of their training...It's a very typical thing I am just starting to (write) now because of my union involvement. The only way you can get things done sometimes if there is a problem, like with nonnursing duties...if people do something that is a nonnursing duty because they have to and there is no one else to do it, they should document it and say "hey look this is taking up x amount of my time" but will they do it? Certainly not in the structured sense. If some-

one sticks a piece of paper on the wall and says "every time you do something that you shouldn't be doing write down what it is and how long it takes and the date." They will do that, they will scribble on the (paper on the) wall, but that's got no credence really. You have got to put it on the official form and write it out in triplicate and all those things, but they won't do it.

Diane took upon herself the task of trying to write up forms on behalf of clinical nurses on nursing issues. However, she found that the administrative processes were lengthy and generally ineffective. These administrative procedures were complex enough to discourage clinical nurses from official complaints enabling the status quo to be maintained. Administrators could argue that they had few documented complaints, and nurses could argue that the procedures were time-consuming and ineffectual. Hegemony was maintained because the clinical nursing culture is based on oral communication, whereas the administrative culture is based on written communication. This written communication is legitimated and afforded hierarchical status over oral communication within the hospital culture. Hegemony is also re-created and maintained by unquestioning acceptance of unexamined behaviors and actions, which have their roots in the socialization practices of the past. An obvious example of this is the routine engaged in by nurses for tea and lunch breaks. The following excerpt comes from a taped discussion with Bev. I was presenting her with my observations, for her responses and reflections, on the tea break ritual (throughout my comments on the tape Bev was nodding and making noises of agreement but for brevity I have omitted them). The tape begins with me presenting my observations for Bev to concur, challenge, change or enlarge upon:

A.S.: In looking at the meaning behind some of the routines I am interested to see instances such as how nurses go to first tea or second tea. I noticed this run around. "First tea" "Who is on First tea? Come on, come on," and then all these nurses would get together and people would say, "don't go without me," and then there would be this rush out the door and someone would say "I have got to go to the toilet, just wait for me," or others would say, "I will be there in a minute, hold the lift," and there would be this wait at the lift...

Bev: Yes yes!

A.S.:   and another would say: "I have got to put a script in," so when they are walking down they want the others to wait at the pharmacy entrance, and then they would all go into the dining room together.

Bev: That's right

A.S.:   That would interest me because I would then get to the dining room and watch people whom I knew were friends with another person sitting at another table—even an adjoining table—and they would wave and say "hi," but they would always sit down with the nurses on their shift—even when they were all a lot of strangers—people that they had never worked with on a shift before. This happens on the wards quite a bit—particularly with people who have just been shifted or work with (the nurse) bank. It happens in Intensive Care too because sometimes I have seen staff from Coronary Care put into Intensive Care when it was busy, and when we went to tea the table of CCU nurses was next to the ICU table. But those nurses would still sit with the ICU nurses despite the fact that all their friends are there on the coronary care table, and they daren't move—especially the women.

Bev: Yes, you're right!

A.S.:   When they are there, they will talk about their diets or what they did last night, or something, because they don't know each other well, and they don't talk much about nursing. It is their break, but because they often don't know each other well, they don't seem to talk much at a relational level. That surprised me as in other female-dominated professions I have observed it is the men who maintain the general conversation and the women who relate more about their lives and their work.

Bev: Yes, that's interesting.

A.S.:   I have also noticed that the male nurses will sometimes go and sit together and don't necessarily sit with their shift, or if they do they tend to sit at the end and get their paper out and ignore the conversation.

Bev: Yes, that's true!

A.S.:   I have noticed this departure routine happening a great number of times, and it seemed to me to be strange because in other professional situations there wouldn't be this kind of dependency on each other at this level—all walk out together, go down the lifts together...

Bev: They wouldn't all be going to the loo together either!

A.S.:   It seems unusual to me not to go and sit and talk with your friends. So I asked the nursing supervisor "why does this happen like this?" and she said: "Oh it's to help build up the team."

Bev: Was she saying that this behavior was intentional?

A.S.:   Yes. She wasn't saying that it was a good thing. She was saying that this is the rationale from the hospital administrators.

Bev: What would admin have to do with that?

A.S.:   Well there is a socialization process at work. Why would everybody do that?

Bev: I don't know.

A.S: Well you think what happened to you in the early days.

At this point Bev began to respond to the data using examples from her own clinical nursing experience to substantiate her reflective process. She demonstrates the potential for the reflective process to uncover habitual ways of thinking and acting and the historical processes that create and constrain hegemony.

Bev: Yes well, I hadn't ever really thought about it, but there are a few things that are jumping to mind from what you have said. I went to lunch just before I left, and in the lift I met my friend who now works as a clinical teacher and we agreed to sit together for lunch. We did all our personal gasbagging as fast as we could as we were walking along, before we actually got to the table, as we knew when we got to the table we wouldn't be able to say what we felt. And then as we walked in there was this dilemma—where do we sit? My friend said, "we had better sit near my mob or I am going to get razzed from all the other people for not sitting with the locals," and I said "fair enough." I couldn't have cared less really except that I was in charge and it is a time to sit down and find out how your staff are. Sometimes you can pick up things at lunch time that you may never know about people. So from that point of view it can be useful, but really that is work and not really relaxing at lunchtime. There is no time to talk to your friends on a personal level...Anyway back to the story...when my friend left early, I got a drink and went to sit with my shift, and they all said: "Oh not sitting with us today weren't you?" So you are right, the pressure is on to sit with them. I remember when I started training people taught us that when we were in the dining room if the director of nursing came in we would have to stand up. And that we should never sit at a particular table as that was administration's table. There used to be separate doctors' and nurses' dining rooms. However, it was never taught as a written rule from administration that you sat at particular table, but you certainly did.

A: It is pretty subtle really because you learnt it quickly without written rules.

As Bev reflected on her professional history she began to identify different hegemonic structures in operation, which produced the same effect of conformity and docility.

Bev: Yes. Now I am thinking about it I remember that at the...hospital when I was training, if there was someone (another student) from your school sitting in the cafeteria you would go and sit with them. In fact we didn't do that—sit together on shifts—we sat with our peers (other students).

A.S.:   Do you think that that country hospital was less regimented?

Bev: Maybe, but when I think about it...if you didn't know
         the registered nurses very well you tended to sit with
         your peers (students) because sometimes you weren't
         invited to sit with them (RNs) and you didn't feel com-
         fortable enough to just go and sit there. Now that's a
         totally opposite thing but it still relates to the dependen-
         cy thing doesn't it?

A.S.: Yes, it seems so to me. I spoke to the ICU charge nurse
         about this, and she asked me "what else do you notice
         about the first shift/second shift thing?" She said "there
         is really no rational reason why nurses should behave
         like that." I told her that I had noticed one thing that to
         me seems strange and that is the way your timing is
         organized.

Bev: It is stupid!

A.S.: Some nurses are in the middle of a procedure and
         another nurse will say "first tea," and they will say to
         the person next to them, "look I haven't finished this, I
         will be back after tea, could you keep an eye on my
         patient," and that nurse could also be in the middle of a
         procedure and then has to walk out of the bay to a posi-
         tion where they can observe both patients, and leave
         two patients half-finished because that first nurse felt
         that they had to walk out the door and go to tea at the
         same time as the others. Anyway, when I reported this
         to the charge nurse, she agreed and said that was what
         she had been concerned about and we talked about
         alternatives. Then she started the new system of making
         independent arrangements with the nurse in the next
         bay so that nurses could decide to go to tea when it was
         convenient for the patients and for the other nurse to
         watch your patient. We thought this would be good
         nursing and would allow people room to escape from the
         dependency thing. But it hasn't happened really.

   Further reflection enabled Bev to recognize the irrational
nature of the habitual routines and modes of behavior and the
strategies used by nurses to resist rational action.

Bev: The other thing with responsibility, too, is that so many
         nurses stick into their bay and not be ready to go to tea

anyway. I know I used to get fed up with that thing of waiting for everyone and I would say "let's go, there's no point waiting because otherwise we would lose half our tea break." But people used to get mad at me for saying that. They were very resistant to going ahead. It was almost like you were being rude to the person that you had to wait for. I mean there was only one thing that I would try and stick by and that was if we were going down to an unusual place for tea and a lot of ICU nurses don't know anyone else from the wards, then from that point of view I wouldn't mind waiting so I could tell people where to go.

A.S.: Oh that's fine. I have really appreciated people taking me with them when I haven't known where to go. I was just surprised that so many people have been unable to do what you suggest and to be able to walk out by the lift and say "I am going to the dining room for tea. See you down there."

Bev: I agree.

A.S.: Then the other nurse can say "I won't be down for five minutes because I won't finish this patient until then, and I will take five minutes extra." So that nurses can take responsibility for themselves, and so there can be some flexibility.

Bev: Yes, I agree.

A.S.: When I talked this over with the charge nurse she said, "it makes so much more sense for people to go when it suits the patient and them, and the nurse who has to watch their bay anyway, than to just go when everyone else goes and even leave an unsafe or unstable situation."

Bev: Yes.

A.S.: But it isn't really working.

Bev: No. I couldn't stand the old situation from the point of view that very often nobody would be watching the nurseless patient. Even though you would ask someone to watch your patient, you would know they wouldn't. And what is worse a lot of times people would go to tea and not even hand over to someone.

This excerpt demonstrates the cultural pressures felt by nurses to maintain routines, which are not beneficial for themselves in terms of personal and professional relationships or for the patients. All the nurses that I spoke to immediately recognized their behaviors in the description of the tea break ritual and talked about how it demonstrated the passivity and insecurity of nurses and the maintenance of the rituals from nursing's cultural legacy. However, most had not previously questioned either the routine, its history, or its consequences for themselves and their patients. The instigation of a changed more rational practice by the charge nurse did not work because it was implemented hierarchically and because it did not address the nurse's needs for companionship and security when entering the large hospital dining room or take account of the role played by embodiment in developing physical responses and needs such as hunger and fatigue. Nurses agreed that the tea break routine was unsatisfactory, but their comments showed that the more rational system, which enabled them to take responsibility for planning their breaks to suit the needs of the patient and the other nurse who would watch their patient, did not meet their emotional and physical needs either:

> I know the new way is better really, but I hate going down to the dining room by myself and thinking where will I sit and who will I sit with. It is OK if you know that there is a group down there, but this way I mightn't know people to sit with. (RN, medical ward)

> I usually go to first tea on an early (shift) as I can't face breakfast at 5:45 a.m., so by first tea I am starving and food is all I can think of. With this new system I have to negotiate with another nurse and sometimes she wants to go to early, too, and if we are busy we don't just leave like we did before. I get so that all I can think of is two dim sims and a cream bun! (RN, ICU)

As a participant-observer I became aware of the role of embodiment in habits and routines when I found my body needs and rhythms were totally out of sympathy with the routines of the nurses. I couldn't face cream buns and dim sims at 9:30 a.m., but I was very hungry and fatigued from standing and walking in confined spaces by 12:30 p.m. and found it very difficult to wait until 1:45 p.m. for lunch and a chance to sit down.

The nurses, like I, had been encultured into routines and habits that affected their bodily functions and needs. This enculturation process was perpetuated and inscribed more deeply in their bodies each day as they acted in the same way. These processes of enculturation and embodiment combined to maintain a hierarchy of power/knowledge, which perpetuated the gap between the the oral clinical culture and the written administrative culture aligning them with the alleged gap between the "doers" (practitioners) and the "thinkers" (educators and administrators).

Nursing Resistance

Clinical nurses are not cultural dopes. They are aware of many of the ways in which they are oppressed, and in many instances they are aware of the ways in which they are implicated in their own oppression and in the oppression of others. This awareness of their own role in the perpetuation and re-creation of clinical and structural practices that are perceived as oppressive has led individuals and groups of nurses to resist them.

Resistance may be passive such as when instructions are ignored or modified, or it may be active when nurses assert themselves to challenge those staff who have power to require them to act in particular ways. Resistance results from an analysis of the situation and a decision to act in a manner that is more liberating for the individual themselves or for others.

The areas in which these nurses are most articulate are the relationships between themselves and the doctors, between themselves and the members of nursing administration, and between themselves and the nurse educators. These relationships are the key areas where their oppression is most explicit and where they are most active in acts of resistance.

Naive Reforming: Prelude to Resistance

During discussions with, and observations of, these nurses, it appears that some of them are working in a way that is best described by Freire's "naive reforming" stage. People who are naive reformers subscribe to the notion that when particular individuals in the present situation are changed or the present system is made to work perfectly, then the oppressive, conflict-producing situations will no longer exist. This stage is characterized by situations where nurses can expend a lot of energy challenging the mechanics of an administrative decision rather than challenging the basis upon which the decision is made. In this way nurses will make decisions to support or hinder particular doctors based on their feelings about, and perceptions of, that particular doctor, rather than challenging the basis of medical domination and the gender issues inherent in the doctor-nurse relationship. Therefore, unpopular doctors are singled out as examples of the role of medical dominator, whereas popular doctors are excused because "he really cares about the patient" or "he listens to you even if he doesn't do what you suggest." This process disguises the inequality of the doctor-nurse relationship and maintains the hegemonic oppressive relationship. This will not change until nurses are able to critically examine the "crucial rules and roles of the system that create unequal power, place people in conflict, and exploit, oppress or hinder their responsible human development" (Alschuler 1986:493).

Nurses in the naive reforming stage maintain a generalized faith in the knowledge and power of the doctors, which informs their relationships with them. Their conflicts with medical decisions do not develop into resistance because they do not analyze and resist the hegemony of medical power/knowledge. The following incident demonstrates the naive reforming stage when an experienced ICU nurse resolved her conflict with a medical decision by valuing medical knowledge over her own clinical knowledge and experience.

> The new doctor asked the nurse to change the settings on the dials of the machine regulating the oxygen flow to the bloodstream of a postoperative cardiac patient. She asked him what he wanted to do. He explained that he wanted to bring more oxygen into his blood even though he knew that this would increase the breathing rate and make him hyperventilate. The nurse argued that the patient's present rate was not excessive and that from her experience of nursing many postoperative cardiac patients, she had found that the patient would stabilize without treatment within an hour whereas remedial treatment meant that

the patient would be dependent on the ICU equipment for much longer.The doctor responded by agreeing that he understood her argument because he had been through it with the previous nurse who had just handed over the patient and as a result of that discussion he had spoken to the senior anaesthetist. He reminded the nurse that he had been given the authority to make the decision. The nurse agreed to change the setting but reminded him that the patient would hyperventilate.

Later, I asked the nurse how she felt about the decision. She said:

Technically he is right. But I have had a lot of experience nursing these patients, and I know that it (the changed setting) is unnecessary because they do stabilize. He doesn't realize this because this is only his second patient here. However, it is his decision because he has to carry the decision legally. The patient isn't at risk but will be uncomfortable longer. The doctors know more about these things than nurses because they spend all those years getting educated and anyway, it is not my responsibility because the doctor holds the legal responsibility for the patients.

In this incident the nurse's clinical knowledge and experience was in conflict with the doctor's orders. When it became obvious that the doctor was determined to change the oxygen level, she made a judgement that this decision would not put the patient at risk and adhered to it. The action of this nurse was consistent with her usual practice when faced with medical directives in areas where she had more knowledge and experience. When questioned on this she would reiterate her belief that "doctors know much more than nurses because they do all that study and anyway its their patient, they have the legal responsibility. He is only a new doctor, he'll learn." Within the doctor-nurse relationship, she devalued her own specific technical and practical knowledge of cardiac patients and their responses to ventilation and accepted the doctor's decision although she knew that it was an application of a classic textbook theory, which was promulgated through his inexperience with cardiac patients. Her recognition of the fact that the doctor would learn through his mistakes demonstrates the cultural legacy of nursing the doctor rather than the patient.

As this nurse had predicted, the patient in this incident did become more distressed with the increased ventilation necessitating the intervention of the unit medical director to reduce the level. Nurses who treat each doctor-nurse conflict as an isolated case and devalue their own clinical knowledge in areas of their specific competence, perpetuate the naive reforming stage rather than developing critiques, which inform acts of resistance aimed at transformation.

Beyond Naive Reforming: Becoming Critical

Alschuler (1986:493) states that in the process of becoming critical, people move from a "position of passivity, pessimism, victimization, and acceptance of the status quo to a role of actively collaborating in actively creating situations that are more just, liberating, and loving." Giroux (1983:110) argues that it is important to analyze all oppositional forms of behavior to see if they constitute a form of resistance and to recognize that resistance is "an analytical construct and mode of inquiry that contains a moment of critique and a potential sensitivity to its own interests." He describes these as an interest in radical consciousness-raising and collective critical action. However, he also argues that all oppositional behavior needs to become a focal point for dialogue and critical analysis. An examination of the evidence that I have collected illustrates this process as a strengthening of the acts of resistance over the acts of accommodation.

It is necessary to examine evidence of oppositional forms of behavior in nursing from the perspectives of resistance to highlight the points at which the hegemonic relationships between doctors and nurses are fragile and, therefore, have the potential to be transformed through the development of a dialogue of protest and emancipatory actions. I have selected some instances from my observations or discussions that range from passive resistance to acts of resistance, which are a specific response to collaborative critique and can be perceived as emancipatory in intent.

Passive Resistance

Passive resistance is particularly evident in the actions of clinical nurses to nursing care plans. Clinical nurses did not consider nursing care plans necessary for clinical nursing perceiving them to be an added burden for already busy nurses to deal with. The nurses in the study did not believe that the nursing notes and care plans were functional and so engaged in passive resistance by either ignoring the charts, making a minimal effort to record information, or by being deliberately absent from the ward or busy with the patient just before the shift ended.

Diane: Nurses don't like writing down what they do. These nursing notes are generally useless. I tend to read the medical notes and don't bother with the nursing notes.

A.S.: So how do you know what nursing care is needed or has been given?

Diane: We hear it in handover. You have plenty of time to talk to the nurse and then you look after the patient when the nurse is having a meal break. Then if you have any questions you can ask the nurse when they come back. We have to write up nursing care plans. The format has been changed three times so far, and all the nurses get fed up. I guess the college-trained nurses will want to write but we don't.

A.S.: J. is college trained, and she is always complaining about them.

Diane: Yes, I guess they only do them when they have to in their training, but when they work on the wards they feel that they are a waste of time.

Nursing administration had attempted to deal with this problem by designing changes to the forms to enable the nurses to fill them in more accurately. However, these changes were seen to be related to things that were important for administration and not for clinical nurses, and so the nurses used the excuse that they didn't understand the new forms as reasons for noncompliance. The poor response to the changed forms concerned senior administrative staff who developed another form with more guidelines. This form was introduced to the wards and ICU units by the clinical nurse teachers attached to those areas. However, these education sessions were poorly attended and also missed the number of nurses who worked

part-time shifts, night shifts, were on leave, on "days off," or
were agency staff. This meant that on any shift it was unlikely
that there were more than two nurses who had any familiarity
with the new forms. Nurses continued to be baffled and resistant to the new care plan forms and to engage in the previously mentioned forms of passive resistance. This process continued during the term of observation when I noted that three
new nursing care plan forms were developed, instigated, and
passively resisted during an eight-month period. The last care
plan was instigated with an emphasis on the possible legal
penalties which could be incurred by nurses if their nursing
activities were not recorded. At this stage nursing care plans
were filled in more regularly but many nurses only wrote
things that they considered could be the subject of legal ramifications. These recordings continued to be retrospective rather
than prospective care plans to be used during the shift and to
contain projections for future care.

Resistance and the Culture of Silence

The doctor-nurse game has received considerable attention in nursing literature since Stein (1967) first described it
(Ashley 1972, Bullough 1975, Chinn 1985). These writings have
uncovered the manipulative practices used by nurses to maintain the myth that the doctor always knows best, by prompting
and providing clues or covering up instances of malpractice.
Speedy (1986:24) claims that these dishonest communication
games maintain the stereotypes of the dominance of the doctor
over the subservient nurse. Maresh (1986) argues that the barriers to the development of nursing as a distinct and comple-
mentary profession to medicine are feminization, a process
which she describes as the systematic socialization into subservience, unquestioning, and passive behaviors; learned helplessness, which arises from powerlessness; hierarchical structures, which place effective power over nurses in the hands of
males; and patriarchal dominance leading to role playing and
stereotyped behavior. According to Anyon (1984), powerless
women will appropriate and use femininity as a form of resistance, and for nurses a conscious use of femininity as a weapon
may be part of the process of achieving appropriate actions by
medical staff for some patients.

My discussions with clinical nurses indicate that the

women's movement has raised their consciousness of themselves as women and the patterns of behavior that they use to
cope with the constant daily reminders of inferior status as
women and as nurses. However, they also argue that there are
few clinical nurse role models for them to work with because
they recognize that many of the senior administrative staff have
become "adapted" in that they have taken on many of the
alleged male characteristics of aggression, exploitation, and
domination to receive a measure of status and control from
senior medical personnel. The work of Freire (1972) is helpful in
understanding the adapted role of senior nursing administrators. He describes the ideological blindness of people who have
been oppressed—a distortion of reality deriving from their
"adherence" to the oppressor. The oppressed do not perceive
themselves as the actors or subjects in their own social drama
but as objects participating in the drama of the oppressors. This
leads to a desire to emulate or identify with the world of the
oppressor. They are unable to perceive the causes of oppression
or the contradictions inherent in an adaption to the status quo.
They participate unknowingly in a "culture of silence."

This culture of silence has important ramifications for
nurses who are attempting to resist the hierarchical power and
technical base of medical decisions. In the following account a
charge nurse challenged the medical director of her area on his
decision to allow extra surgery when she did not have the necessary bed or staff to cope. She described the situation.

> I believe that medicine and nursing are different, and that
> decisions that affect the running of the ward should be
> made in consultation with me as head nurse. The medical
> director had made a decision to do more surgery because
> it brings in more money to the unit, but you can't make
> medical decisions in isolation from nursing decisions.
> Medical decisions about surgery are based on the needs of
> the patient before surgery, on the availability of theater
> staff and on an projected length of stay in hospital. How-
> ever, not all patients heal at the same rate or come into
> surgery in an ideal condition, so nursing decisions are
> based on the nursing support needed for the patients
> already in the unit, on their actual stay in hospital, on the
> number of beds available, and the number of experienced
> nursing staff available in the unit. When I explained this

to him, he was angry. He reminded me that he was in charge of the whole unit. I told him that I believed that the head nurse had parity with the head doctor and that I had the responsibility for the nursing service and patient care. He didn't accept that I was on a par with him of course so he went to the medical superintendent who went to the director of nursing and I got hauled over the coals. But the doctor didn't go ahead with the extra surgery. It's all political. When the doctors don't get their way they go over our heads to the medical superintendent who goes to the nursing administration. I find that on issues like this, they always support the doctors rather than us.

This nurse has a very clear understanding of her nursing role as distinct from, and equal with, medical practitioners. However, her understanding is not shared by the doctors who see themselves as holding a dominant role, a view which is shared and supported by adapted nursing administrators, who take punitive action in support of the doctor's claims to supremacy. Her resistance could be described as an emancipatory action because she spoke out to protect the quality of care for her patients and as an advocate for the nurses on her staff.

The clinical nurses in the research recognize and reject the models provided by these adapted leaders who discriminate against them in the female-dominated, male-subjugated world of hospital nursing. They recognize that these women can be seen to have identified with masculine traits and participate in competitive behavior that often consists of vertical and horizontal violence. Freire (1972) argues that this horizontal violence is symptomatic of the behavior of members of oppressed groups who become alienated from each other and deflect the violence away from the powerful oppressor to another powerless person.

Diane discussed her experience of horizontal violence at a hospital meeting of RANF members. The members had been asked to discuss whether they were prepared to support the Gippsland nurses who were on strike.

When the issue of the striking nurses was raised there was a big reaction. It was amazing. Since the strike many nurses have felt incredibly guilty and so when they heard of more industrial action there was an emotional response from our nurses who are a nonpolitical middle-class group. The anger was phenomenal. It was the first time that I have seen real union bashing from our members. Nurses were screaming across the room to each other. They weren't listening or thinking. They were all on their own guilt trips.

Horizontal violence is not confined to nurses. Resident doctors often feel powerless in the face of demands and expectations of senior consultants and engage in horizontal violence directed towards senior nursing staff. Observing Eve, I noticed that when a resident had been corrected by the consultant in front of Eve and myself, he became angry. Later when there was a query about some bruising under the arms of a patient, the resident suggested to the consultant that it was the result of injections given by nurses.

Eve: The bruising wouldn't be from injections.

Doctor: Well the nursing staff give the injections.

Eve: Not under the arms!

Dr: With the nursing staff here nothing surprises me.

Accommodation and Resistance as a Simultaneous Process

The nurses in the study are critical of feminists who are writing about how nursing roles should develop without being active participants in clinical nursing. They see them as setting standards and expectations for clinical nurses from the relative safety of academia. This could be seen as an example of the horizontal violence being done to clinical nurses by others who shape their critique far from the realities of the bedside. Speedy (1986:26) describes Heide as a tireless activist for feminism and nursing before going on to explain that she had to leave nursing or else "suffer psychologically." Many of these critiques imply that the only response to the stereotypic doctor-nurse role is acceptance or rejection. The evidence that I have collected reflects a range and diversity of reactions that can be described as a "simultaneous process of accommodation and resistance" (Anyon 1984:24). Nurses are not social-

ized into passively receiving a stereotyped role; the socialization process is one of actively responding and reacting to the
contradictions inherent in doctor-nurse roles and relationships. This simultaneous process of accommodation and resistance was evident during an observation session of Bev. She
found herself in exactly the same situation as the nurse mentioned previously who exemplified naive reforming.

> Bev had set the ventilator to the low level that her experi-
> ence suggested was appropriate for the patient. A new
> surgical intern came into the bay and began fiddling with
> the dials on the ventilator. Bev asked him what he wanted
> to do. He ignored her and finally set the ventilator to a
> high setting. She asked why he had changed the setting,
> and he told her that it was safer to provide more oxygen
> initially and that the level could be reduced later. She
> explained why she had set it on the lower setting, but the
> intern reminded her that the patient is "my patient." Bev
> agreed to leave the setting for the moment, but she sug-
> gested that they review the decision when she had taken
> the next set of blood gases (to determine how much oxy-
> gen was getting into the blood stream). Although she
> decided that the patient was not at risk with the higher
> setting, she told me that she was concerned that the
> patient would be rather uncomfortable as a result of the
> inexperience of the intern. As she was a senior nurse and
> the intern was a junior doctor, she decided to go over his
> head, and when he had left the bay, she called the senior
> anaesthetist on another pretext and then casually men-
> tioned: "We are maintaining the patient on level 10."
>
> As she had predicted the senior doctor replied: "Oh well,
> we can put him on 4 now don't you think."
>
> The nurse readily agreed and he changed the level. When
> the intern returned and queried the change she told him
> that the senior anaesthetist had changed the levels when
> he came into the bay.

In this incident the nurse judged her role to be an advocate
for the comfort of her critically ill patient. When her initial resistance had not led to success, she accommodated to the wishes
of the doctor and then she resorted to manipulation of both doc-

tors to achieve her goal for her patient. In a subsequent discussion on this incident she agreed that she had been manipulative but felt that although she had a lot of credibility with the senior medical staff in the unit, if she had asked the intern to come with her to jointly discuss it with the senior anaesthetist, then the senior doctor would have sided with the junior doctor. She felt that manipulation was the only form of resistance open to her other than accommodation in her powerless position.

Resistance: Collective Critique in Action

Resistance develops as a group of people engage in a process of enlightenment through ideology critique and act upon this enlightenment to empower and emancipate others. The most effective acts of resistance were the result of a collective engagement in a critique of the situation, which led to a communal consciousness raising. Individuals were empowered by this collaborative critique to resist oppressive situations and become effective advocates for their patients. This was evident in situations such as the following.

> I was following Eve as she went on a round with the resident, intern, and consultant.The round was about to pass a patient who had been in ICU for a long time. After initial medical treatment he had remained in ICU for specialist nursing care. As he was not receiving active medical treatment I had noticed that the doctors round would not even stop and check on his progress. On this day Eve asked that the doctors check his progress as the nursing staff felt that he no longer needed intensive nursing care and could be moved to a ward. The doctors disagreed and said that as he had a trachy in he was not ready to leave ICU. In her words:
>
>> That made me mad. They had been skipping on the round for so long that they had no current knowledge about him. We had all worked really hard to get him ready for the ward.
>
> The consultant then told Eve that the ward hadn't been able to manage him before.
>
> Eve: Yes, that is because of his trachy. We think that he is ready to have his trachy out.

C: No, I don't agree with you.

Eve: Then could you give me the indications that mean
       that the trachy should remain in.

The consultant then examined the patient and agreed that
he was unable to give her good reasons why the trachy
should remain in. He asked her to tell him why she
thought the patient would be able to function on the
ward. Eve explained all the reasons why the nursing staff
believed that he should go to the ward.

C: All right, have what you want.

The consultant then strode quickly to the next bay and
turned to Eve and said pointedly: "Before we start, is
there anything *you* want to say about *this* patient?"

Critiques of the organization of nursing practices can
unearth the power base upon which they have been developed.
Practices can be identified as being instigated in the interests
of the doctors, the administrators, or even the nurses rather
than in the interests of the patients. When the interests of the
patient becomes the focus, practices can be resisted and
restructured to support quality patient care as evident in these
comments from Eve:

When I arrived the patients charts were all kept in the doctor's office. The nurses had to go there all the time to fill in
the information. This meant that they had to leave their
critically ill patients and then interrupt doctors and excuse
themselves to get to the files. I wanted the nurses caring
for their patients at the bedside not getting caught up in
the doctor's office, so we all (nurses) discussed this problem, and I told the doctors that I wanted all patient information to be held at the bedside so that the nurses had
access to it as a basis for their decisions about patient
care. The doctors weren't happy about it, so I suggested
that if they wanted to keep control over the files then they
should do the procedures (blood tests, etc.) themselves
and write them up. Of course, they didn't want to do that,
so now we have all the charts at the bedside.

This new arrangement not only allowed the nurses continual access to important patient information to inform their clin-

ical judgements but enabled the doctors and paramedics to check the information and see the patient at the same time rather than arriving at the bedside with sketchy notes to support their memories.

Resistance: An Engagement in a Transformative Process

Resistance to oppressive situations, which results in transformative actions, is generally not the brief process depicted in the previously reported examples. In instances where nurses are intent on transforming a situation in which they are relatively powerless in the face of rampant bureaucracy, they may be engaged in a long process of resistance with a variety of representatives from departments.

Carol recounted her experience of a long process of resistance in order to bring about a transformation of intolerable conditions for patients.

> When you work in a hospital, you find that no one will make a decision. No one will definitely say "yes." You have to deal with invisible people. It is so hard to get a decision because it needs to be authorized by "they" whoever "they" are. We have memo warfare with anonymous people. It is crazy to expect that to achieve anything because you can never find the mysterious " they" who have the power. When the official channels break down, then you start the informal strategies. After doing this a few times, the official channels get a token memo and you go straight to the informal channels. That's OK if you or your supervisor have been around the hospital for a time and know all the different people, but if you are new I don't know how you can get much done. If you know people you can sometimes approach them directly and arrange for them to come and do something and then report back to whichever "they" look after that area. Sometimes that works, but you need friends in high places if you want to make big changes.

Carol is describing the structured resistance inbuilt in bureaucratic organizations. Nurses are particularly disadvantaged in these situations because their work is organized around shifts that don't regularly coincide with the working

hours of those who work within the administration and maintenance departments of the hospital. Nurses, such as Carol, need
a considerable amount of time and patience to engage in the
kind of structured acts of resistance that lead to transformations in the situations experienced by their staff and patients.

> I was really mad about the air conditioning. This building
> was designed with all this glass facing west into the sun
> so it would get really hot in the rooms, especially the
> small rooms. I used to complain, and the engineers would
> come and take the temperature from the main desk in the
> cool part of the ward and then report that it was the right
> temperature. We finally took the temperatures of the win-
> dows and the metal was really hot, between 30–40
> degrees centigrade, and so were the patients near them.
> We had to wait for over a year for some action. Then we
> had blinds made for the windows and when they arrived
> three months later they didn't fit and we had to use them
> in other rooms that weren't facing the sun and didn't real-
> ly need them.

> Later we had trouble because the air conditioning got so
> cold in winter with all the glass. We had the patients all
> rugged up, and we were all shivering. Patients were get-
> ting hypothermic so we had to drag their beds out into the
> corridor to nurse them. We got a petition with 360 signa-
> tures. It took ages to get action on that. We used to put
> brown paper bags over the vents because they were all
> situated directly above the patient's beds. They would be
> lying in bed with six blankets and still be cold. It took us
> two years to get that air conditioning changed.

Carol's final reflection highlights the manner in which
technologies of power combine to develop docility in nurses
leading to apathy and a perpetuation of hegemony through a
denial of the opportunity to reflect on their clinical practice.

> When you spend so much time getting things right that
> should never have been wrong in the first place, then you
> don't have the opportunity to think about other things.

Acts of resistance to the hegemony of oppressive situations can bring about transformation. These transformative

acts are directed towards enlightenment, empowerment, and emancipation from oppression in all its forms and structures. As nurses continue to critique medical domination, administrative structures, gender politics, and the legacy of nursing culture, they will continue to uncover the hierarchies of power/knowledge that oppress their clinical knowledge and practice. The valuing of the power of clinical knowledge leads to critiques on patient care and the values that shape and govern the way in which technical knowledge is legitimized by doctors, administrators, paramedics, and nurses.

13

❧

If I Knew More I Could Do More

A common complaint among nurses is the fact that they are lacking information about the ways in which decisions are made by the medical staff, nursing administration, and their nursing colleagues. This complaint evidences testimony to the adage attributed to Francis Bacon, "Knowledge itself is power." Foucault (1972) writes of the interrelationships between power and knowledge disclosing the manner by which power constitutes knowledge, and knowledge constitutes power. He highlights the essential interrelatedness of power and knowledge in his concept of power/knowledge.

Power/Knowledge as an Analytical Construct

Power/knowledge is a valuable analytical concept because it enables nurses to uncovers historical constructions in nursing practice, the values inherent in nursing knowledge and practices, the interests being served by the maintenance of the hegemonic situations, and the contradictions inherent in nursing theory and nursing practice. These understandings form the basis for critique, contestation, and resistance leading to transformative action. It was apparent from the case record that the nursing strike had radicalized many nurses, and some of these were attempting to make changes to transform situations that demonstrated injustice and inequity. The most successful transformative actions came about when individual nurses were able to make a difference in the life of an individual patient.

Power/Knowledge and Temporality

Nurses who were able to locate their patients within an understanding of temporality were able to use their clinical judgement to determine the needs of the patient at a particular point in the healing or dying process and understand this in relation to the particular patient's past health situation and their expected future movement through the healing or dying process. The capacity to assess the patient as a product of their own personal health history and to make informed projections about future health needs and care is developed through reflection upon the previous clinical experiences and knowledge of the nurse. It is evident in the act of connoisseurship in the nursing care given by Carol to a frail patient who was obviously trying to hide her fears about her illness and the future.

> During the drug round Carol spent time speaking to each patient. She was particularly concerned that a female patient, "Mary," was unable to get enough pain relief and to sit or lie comfortably in or out of bed and sat and talked with her. Carol explained that she was reluctant to suggest to the doctors that Mary be given a higher dosage of painkillers as they were making her feel ill and she was not eating. Mary was extremely thin, and it was difficult for her to get comfortable because of pain in her ribs.

During this discussion Carol was ascertaining the extent of Mary's medical problem in relation to her overall needs. She chooses to engage in some practical help aimed at making the patient more comfortable.

> After the drug round, Carol went and found the physiotherapist and talked with her about Mary's discomfort. The physio went and spent time with the patient before coming back to Carol and telling her that she felt that Mary needed to be seated in a more comfortable chair with something soft and supportive around her back. The physio reported that she had tried to sit the patient in a lounge chair with extra cushions but that it was the wrong shape for the patients. Carol suggested that they try sitting Mary in a bean bag. We took the bean bag into the ward, and Carol explained to the patient that we were

proposing to sit her in it while she ate her lunch. The patient was a little alarmed at first but responded to Carol's reassurances that it was only a trial and she didn't have to use it if it was no good for her. Carol got me to shape up the bag and give demonstrations of how to sit in it. Then I shook the bag again and the physio and a young work experience student lifted the frail woman into the bag. Unfortunately she was not heavy enough to make a shape and too sore to wriggle in it, so she was lifted back on to the bed,and I was delegated to sit in it and wriggle to make the appropriately shaped hole. The patient was lifted down again but appeared very anxious. Carol squatted down beside her and said "Now Mary are you uncomfortable being so close to the floor?" Mary nodded. Carol continued: "Well no wonder you can see under your bed and under all these other beds in the ward. That's no good."

So we moved her back on her bed, and Carol sat with her holding her hand and asked her if she would like to try once again with the bean bag placed on her lounge chair to give her height and support. Mary agreed to try again so we repeated the routine with me preparing the seat by sitting in it and wriggling down and the physio and assistant lifting the patient into it. It was obvious that the patient was too fragile to move at all to make her self comfortable in the bean bag so I helped the physio lift her back into bed. The patient was very apologetic. Carol understood what she was feeling and said,

Now Mary you are worried that you have let us down aren't you (Mary nodded). Well, of course you haven't. We were only trying to make you comfortable so that you could eat some lunch. It doesn't matter to us if you sit in the bean bag or on the bed or on the chair. We just want you to be comfortable. We didn't know if that would work or not. We are just glad that you tried it. Now I will leave you to have a rest and put on my thinking cap and see if there is some other way to help you get comfortable because I am worried that you are in pain and not able to eat properly.

Carol then spoke with the doctor and arranged for a new drug regime to help the patient with pain control. Although

Carol recognized that physical comfort was the first priority for this patient, she acted as an interpreter of Mary's needs and feelings and as an advocate on Mary's behalf with the physiotherapist and doctor in order to transform Mary's situation. She was prepared to focus on Mary's problem and to obtain a bean bag from a staff room in an attempt to make Mary more comfortable. She had never tried to sit a patient in a bean bag in the ward before but knew that they were used in geriatric nursing homes. During the process Carol was constantly attempting to understand the current situation from Mary's viewpoint as was evident in her understanding of Mary's reluctance to sit where she was looking under beds. She was able to assess that this was a cause for concern by squatting beside Mary and seeing what she saw whereas the physiotherapist was trying to assess Mary's problem from a situation of standing above her. Carol's advocacy role developed when she called for the doctor and insisted that he review all of Mary's medical history and the particular drug regime, which was making her sick. Carol evaluated Mary's unique responses to her health problems in order to transform Mary's fears and subsequent dependence on the nursing staff and the relative safety of the hospital ward to a perspective of confidence in her ability to manage her health problems and become as independent as possible. To achieve this Carol needed to stabilize Mary's condition and to help her see a future beyond the ward and its facilities. In order to do this Carol engaged in a long-term process of transforming Mary's fears into confidence. Five days later I recorded the following interaction between Carol and Mary.

10:45 a.m.:   Carol went to speak with Mary, the patient that she had previously tried to sit out in the bean bag.

C: Hello Mary, what lovely flowers! Did you friend bring them in from your garden?

M: Yes, they are lovely aren't they. They come from our garden.

C: Are we controlling your pain better?

M: Yes, well almost...it's better.

Carol then reviewed M's chart with the RN and checked the new drug regime.

C: How well do you think you are coping? Are you able to get out of bed by yourself?

Mary described the manner which she had devised to enable her to move independently from bed to chair.

C: Good. Well, when do you think that you will be ready to go home?

P: Oh I don't know...I don't think I can say...

M: We are not trying to push you out, but I just want to think about how we are going in relation to getting you home...If we have the district nurse and the O.T. come to assess what aids you could have in your home to help you and if we have your pain under control so that you can look after it yourself, do you think you will be ready to go home soon?

M: Yes...but I don't want to go and then come back again.

C: Well what if we say next Tuesday. That's a week from today. We could send you home for two days and see how you do. In the middle of the week there is the district nurse, the O.T. and home help available.

M: We have the home help come.

C: Yes, well you could have meals on wheels or does your friend like to cook.

M: Yes she makes a hot meal at night...sometimes she cooks the meal for me, and when we are ready to eat I just can't.

C: That worries you doesn't it?

M: Yes, I feel bad that she is so concerned about me...that she has to do so much...she never says anything...never complains, but I worry about her.

C: Well you will have to stop worrying about making your friend worry about you because it just makes a viscous circle...you worry about her and she worries about you worrying about her and it goes on and on. What if we try to organize for you to go home next Tuesday...if you feel up to it. It doesn't matter if you aren't we can easily change the day...but if you have two days at home and you are all right we can discharge you from home. If not we will keep your bed and you can come back. I will be here on Sunday and we will sit down and have a talk about what you think you will do when you can't manage at home because I know that is worrying you.

M: (tentatively) Yes...it is...I do worry about that...My friend won't be able to cope with me forever.

C: Well, we will talk about that on Sunday when we have more time and you are feeling stronger. You are looking better.

M: Yes, I do feel better.

Carol is providing specific goals for Mary to aim at while constantly reassuring her that they are flexible. She is also working to help Mary to face and manage both her short-term fears concerning going home and her long-term fears of the inability of her friend to look after her anymore. This kind of transformative action by clinical nurses occurs regularly although these instances of practice are not recorded or shared with other nurses. They are recorded only as changes to drug regimes on medical and nursing charts, and therefore other nurses are unable to learn from the these kind of examples of clinical expertise.

Although many nurses engage in individual transformative actions with individual patients, most nurses disregard the power/knowledge relations present in the structures and practices in clinical nursing. An effect of horizontal violence has been to isolate nurses from other nurses and reduce their potential for engaging in collaborative critique as a basis for the transformation of oppressive structures for their patients and the enlightenment, empowerment, and emancipation of themselves.

The nurses in this study all engaged in attempts to facilitate structural changes in order to improve conditions that were oppressive and replace them with practices that were more rational. These were individualized attempts to change the structural inequalities inherent in the current nursing situation, which were developed and implemented hierarchically.

These nurses expressed discouragement with the failure of these more rational changes and the capacity of nurses to continue to maintain practices and structures about which they complained almost daily. This frustration was expressed by many nurses in response to the constant problems associated with rosters and shift work.

Rosters are a common problem for all nurses in all wards because shift work affects the social and physical lives of people. Nurses reported having difficulties in sustaining personal relationships through the consequences of working when others were available for leisure activities and of having poor reactions to the disruptions of bodily rhythms through night shifts or constant late/early shifts changes. A number of nurses felt that their professional skills were undermined through poor physical responses to particular shift patterns. Therefore, the fitting together of shift patterns, which suited individual's physical and social needs while providing appropriate coverage for wards in terms of differing levels of seniority and equity of distribution, was a constant challenge for nurses. During the course of this study, roster problems formed a constant theme for discussion resulting in the introduction of self-rostering. This was a rational attempt to enable nurses to negotiate their shift allocations to enable more equitable arrangements. However, the implementation of self-rostering met with considerable resistance for a number of reasons. According to Carol, nurses are conservative and unwilling to take the responsibility to engage in structural change despite their dissatisfactions:

> Junior graduates complain about self-rostering when they go to a ward because then if they make a mistake they have no one to blame. They find it difficult to take the blame for their own mistakes. Nurses are very conservative. They are not given a lot of responsibility in their training, and even with the training going to colleges they come back to work on wards that have a structure, different levels of nurses, rosters, uniforms, shifts, and other things that are part of the nursing tradition. The nurses accept this, and then it is very difficult to bring about change. This applies to things like changing the hours even though nurses complain about their shifts all the time. I tried to introduce a change in the hours on one ward when I was in charge. I had thought it out carefully

and tried to rationalize the hours so that the nursing staff would have more leisure. One or two were happy to try it, but the rest wouldn't. They were so conservative and wanted things to go on the same even though my new plan was more rational. Then they still go on complaining about the hours.

Carol highlights her experience of the hegemony of nursing culture and the apathy towards change that it perpetuates. She also demonstrates the difficulties of attempting to resist irrational practices through hierarchical imposition. The theoretical justification for self-rostering was that it would enable nurses to meet their own needs and the needs of other nurses through a process of negotiation for their shifts. The difficulties in its introduction were often blamed on the nurses themselves rather than the method of introduction. Therefore, a potentially empowering strategy is imposed upon the nurses who would benefit from its adoption. This method perpetuates the situation where nurses are expected to accept structures developed *for* them rather than *with* them. A discussion with Bev demonstrates the consequences of the hierarchical imposition of a strategy, which is aimed at liberating people through negotiation.

Bev: With self-rostering you are supposed to fit around each other, but one nurse used to put in her roster, regardless of what others were requesting, and then someone else would have to come along and juggle it...she wouldn't work it out with the other untrained people. I said, "look all you untrained people you can't be on together, so you just have to get together and work it out." The self-rostering didn't get off to a good start. The charge nurse didn't explain it properly at the start, so it hasn't worked.

A.S.: When I observed a nurse putting down all the weekends off, I asked her did she have something on each weekend and she said she didn't but that she put them all down because she was scared that she won't get any and that she might need them. So she put them all down just in case. I said to her, "If you get all those it means that someone else isn't going to get a free weekend" and she said, "I won't get them all, I just put them in on the off chance that I will get some." And I said, "wouldn't it be more sensible to put down the ones that you really want so that you can be sure that you will get them?" She said, "I don't know."

Bev: Yes. Self-rostering is shot down in flames by the nurses. I wasn't there on the explanation. I came back in and no one talked to the people who didn't understand or who had missed out on the meeting. No one who understood it was delegated to explain it to those who missed out. It was a big change. People were resistant to it. It came at a time of lots of big changes. People are very protective of their rosters. When I came in, I didn't know what it was; I read it and tried to understand it. I thought, "well I think that makes sense," but I had a lot of "what if's" and wondered how it was going to work. I saw the numbers, thought that was fine, generally picked it up, but it was still pretty confusing to me.

A.S.: It is fairly complicated isn't it?

Bev: Yes, it is complicated. Now that was me. I am sure a few of the people had the same feelings. Some would have understood it less. Maybe some read it and understood it better because of past experience. But it was typical of the way senior staff brings in changes. There was no room for an education program. It was brought in too soon. They should have said, "in four weeks time we are going to start self-rostering with the roster going up in two weeks." The change was too rapid without enough warning or consultation, so now people are feeling "oh well, self-rostering doesn't work, so I will have to look after myself, so I will put down every weekend possible."

Bev's comments demonstrate the futility of attempting to empower people without engaging them in the negotiation of the problem and allowing them to develop collaboratively agreed upon strategies for change. Nurses have learned to distrust structures that are hierarchically implemented because they have learned through experience that these strategies rarely empower them. Therefore, when strategies are specifically aimed at empowerment, such as self-rostering and negotiated tea breaks, clinical nurses continue to distrust changes in practices that they do not "own" through a process of problem posing and problem solving. They resist these practices in ways that not only maintain oppression but actually create greater inequity and disadvantage. Bev talks further about the inability of nurses who have been powerless to take empowering opportunities when they are available.

> This is what I mean about whinging and powerless. One of the nurses is always whinging about her roster. So I tried to help her. I haven't got the power to change them so I talked to her about talking to the charge nurse. She told me that she can't talk to her when she is working because she is too busy. So I suggested that she make a time after her shift but she said that she needed to pick up her kids. So then I suggested she make an appointment on her day off but she said she didn't like to go near the hospital on her day off. So I got mad with her. I told her if she wasn't willing to do something about her predicament, no one else was going to help. I said, "Why don't you do something to help yourself?" And she left. Well that's sad that we lost a staff member, but she wasn't willing to negotiate.

The "touristy nurse" is a name coined to describe the high mobility of nurses who tend to move on looking for better conditions rather than attempting to facilitate transformations in those situations which they find intolerable. These nurses eventually leave nursing, and as a result nursing in Victoria is facing a chronic shortage of experienced clinical nurses. This shortage means that is it easy for nurses to continue to move on to other vacancies rather than stay and confront inequities for themselves or their patients.

This confrontation would need to be a collaborative exercise enabling nurses to jointly critique the values implicit in unexamined nursing practices and structures by disclosing the mechanisms of false consciousness as the basis for resistance and transformative action. According to Carol, nurses contribute to their own powerlessness and inability to make emancipatory changes on behalf of their patients by their lack of cohesion.

> They focus on getting their work done. They don't focus on what would be the best for the patients in the long term; they are too busy in the present. If the environment

is unsatisfactory nurses may grumble about it, but they don't think that they can change it. I remember when the new building was built and I saw the ward design. I was amazed and horrified at that rabbit warren that was supposed to be a ward. All those little rooms separate from the others, the positioning of the toilets, the front desk in the middle of the thoroughfare. I couldn't believe it. But people accepted it. If all the charge nurses had combined, they could have changed things, but they just accepted it.

Power/Knowledge and Space

The hospital administration had given the design of the new wards to a firm of architects who did not consult with the people who spend all their working time in the ward providing patient care. Architectural and administrative power/knowledge was considered superior to clinical nursing knowledge in the determination of the best environment in which to provide quality patient care. The ward design reflected aesthetic and administrative values rather than the provision of a health-enhancing environment for patients and a flexible environment that encouraged nurses to engage in imaginative, patient-focused nursing.

Observations of nurses at work indicated that they used the spaces in the wards differently to other staff members and patients. Designers formed spaces with considerations such as accessibility for cleaning or visibility of the nurse's station for other staff and visitors. These considerations meant that although the work of the nurses was visible to others, the patients were scattered through rooms of various sizes separated by corridors and storage places and so were less visible to the nurses. Nurses were separated from each other and rarely had enough room around a bed to provide the patient with the dignity of sufficient privacy. The consequences of this enforced segregation of nurses meant that nurses did not see their own work as part of the contribution of the nursing team to patient welfare and developed as individualists. This individualism was apparent in the distribution of work and in the maintenance of high stress levels. Carol claimed:

I often find that the senior staff on the ward are the worst because when they get overworked they won't ask for help. This happens even when there are nurses near them who are not busy. They just get resentful and let it show. I tell them that they must ask for help as people are not going to keep coming to them to say, "what can we do to help you?" They have difficulty because they are not mature enough to know when to ask for help and how to do it. Many of them have an individualistic approach. They have difficulty thinking that they are part of a team. They think about "their" patients and "their" work and have trouble working together.

Nurses with an individualistic approach claim a symbolic ownership of symbolic spaces. Nurses allocated a number of patients and a physical space in which to engage in patient care treat patients, and the activities which they perform for them, as part of their ownership of clinical nursing in a particular space. Nursing within symbolic space means that nurses can claim to be patient-focused by taking responsibility for all patient care within their allocated space but in effect be only meeting their own needs to do their work for their patients. A patient-centered approach could mean that a busy, stressed nurse with a heavy case load would ask another nurse who is not busy to help her provide quality patient care.

Time/Space and Tasks

Clinical nursing is carried out in the public sphere in a role that of necessity must be responsive to interruptions and rapid changes in their clinical situation. Nurses who think in terms of the workload within symbolic spaces develop habitual routines to achieve their nursing tasks within the shift. Inexperienced nurses rapidly learn to structure their workload in order that they can respond to interruptions or emergencies, by setting time-based lists of tasks in their heads and attempting to be ahead of their planned routines. Therefore, nurses often speak of "getting ahead," or "going well today," or "way behind." The ability to structure the time/space grid within the workload is an important part of learning to be a nurse. However, a consequence of learning to negotiate the time/space grid as an individualist rather than as a team member is the development and consolidation of task-based approaches to nursing.

When the power/knowledge construct overlaps the time/

space construct, it is possible to recognize that the replacement of task allocation with patient allocation or primary care, a theory beloved of nurse educators, will not necessarily bring about enlightenment, empowerment, or emancipation for either the patient or the nurse. The hegemony of the technical approach to patient care reinforces the alienation of the nurse from the painful experiences being undergone by the patient. Nurses operating from a technical base to clinical nursing can learn about Kubler-Ross's (1969) stages of grief and identify with them from their own personal and clinical experiences, but then transform the emancipatory intent of the grief stages into a set of tasks for the patient to complete. Therefore, because these nurses experienced enlightenment and empowerment in their nursing through the "aha" experiences of having their personal and clinical knowledge and experience named and identified by Kubler-Ross, they wanted all their patients to experience this same process of emancipation. However, the power/knowledge of the nursing tradition of reducing theory to a set of tasks to be achieved means that the potentiality of the transformative agenda to enable people to understand their experiences of grief from within a nonprescriptive, broad-based theory developed from experiences, is lost and replaced by a prescriptive, technical application of knowledge. Comments from my notes suggest that this technical application of an empowering theory is relatively common:

> Charge nurse: That man really needs to be made to come and see his wife now, or he may have difficulties in the grief process.

> New graduate to experienced RN: I don't know what to do with Mr G because I can't decide if he is in "denial" or "anger."

> RN to me: Mrs. H is in "denial," but we need to move her along a bit so that she gets through all the stages before she dies.

These comments demonstrate the embedded nature of the technical construction of nursing knowledge. Power/knowledge identifies the historical and technical constructions of nursing culture by which the patient becomes an object to be put through a process by the nurse rather than an active subject collaborating with the nurse and others in experiencing their own unique expression of grief, a process that may be identified in relation to, or informed by, the observations of grieving as described by Kubler-Ross and others.

Therefore, power/knowledge facilitates the identification of embedded values, which inform nursing culture and which can transform emancipatory processes and structures into technical constructions.

Limits to Power/Knowledge

Fay (1987) argues that the specific agenda of enlightenment, empowerment, and emancipation of critical social science, with its acceptance of the value of intersubjective meaning and the potentialities of ideology critique, rational reflection, resistance, and collaboratively determined transformative action, is limited in a number of ways. Therefore, although Fay subscribes to a emancipatory agenda of critical social science, he suggests that there are limits to rationality, clarity, and autonomy. The research process demonstrated the limitations of power/knowledge as a theoretical and analytical tool for nursing.

Limit to Power/Knowledge:
Positive Experiences of Nursing Culture

Clinical nursing does not occur in a time/space vacuum. It is embedded in traditions, historical constructions, and a specific nursing culture. This culture daily shapes nurses and is reciprocally shaped by them. People are attracted to nursing because of this culture and not in spite of it. The positive experiences of nurses engaged in clinical nursing practice reinforce their commitment to nursing and to a maintenance of the nursing culture.

> ...I think I am a good ICU nurse. I don't see my role to represent nursing in the future. I just do a good job here. I think that you can do a lot of talking without getting any good done. (RN, ICU)

> I know that some nurses want to change everything, but I have found that most nurses are like me. We came into nursing because we liked it as it is. I don't mean that

everything is perfect, but there are always hassles in any job. You just take the good with the bad. It worries us that nursing is becoming so academic that people like us would never get accepted in, and yet I think I am a pretty good nurse. (RN, medical ward.)

These attitudes were commonly expressed because within the constraints and oppression of nursing practice, all nurses engage in transformative actions. These transformative actions may relate to their role as interpreter of the hospital and medical problem or situation in a way that enlightens patients to make informed choices or to understand and adjust to changed situations. Bev described her experience as an interpreter of the medical jargon and procedures.

Then you have the...problem with the medicos of when they are trying to communicate to patients, and to nurses, but not so much,...to break it down to language that everyone can understand. It is hard. They can't let go of the technical language...I have many a time witnessed an examination of a patient and they (doctor) will describe what happened and what operation it was and the classic one I remember was the description of an aneurysm repair. The doctor explained this wonderful thing that happened to this man with his arms flailing everywhere and the patient was just captivated by this performance and so were the relatives, and a few comments were made after he left about what a bit of a dag he was, and I said "well did you understand what he said?" They said "no" and looked perplexed. They did not have a clue. I got the pen and the paper out, and I drew it all and showed them what had happened and what the result of it would be. "Oh right" they said in amazement. They had absolutely no idea. I mean he started off with "aorta." Well, they didn't have a clue what an aorta was so they were lost after that, completely lost. So they didn't understand any of the things he said about complications or the implications for his future lifestyle or anything.

Nurses recognize the value of their clinical skills, knowledge, experiences, and relationships when they are participating in the process of transformation of a person from illness to

health or from illness to death. When Bev was a student psychiatric nurse, she was able to critique the effect of medical jargon
on the potentiality of nursing. She found that psychiatric nurses were using medical jargon in nursing notes, and although
she knew that she had unquestioningly accepted medical jargon when working in an ICU ward in a general hospital, the
changed setting and the process of researching her own practice led her to challenge the value of medical jargon for nurses.

> At present I am not caught up in the medical jargon, and I
> don't know if it changes when you become trained...When
> patients say things like "I hate being in hospital; I want to
> go home; I don't know why I should be here; I want to go
> home," then a registered psychiatric nurse will write "lack
> of insight"...lack of insight being medical jargon. What the
> hell can we do about "lack of insight"? Not a thing! What
> we can do something about is the distress caused by not
> wanting to be in hospital. I can. I can make it more inter-
> esting. I can explain the reason why it is reality-based. I
> can do all those kind of things. That's stuff I can do. But I
> can't do anything about lack of insight.

Bev is able to challenge the psychiatric jargon adopted by
psychiatric nurses and to affirm her own practical knowledge
and use it to transform the situation and the patient's understandings. Bev was affirming her ability as a nurse to engage
in interpretive and transformative actions on behalf of her
patients. She was recognizing the uniqueness of her contribution to patient welfare.

Although nurses expressed their feelings of inadequacies,
uncertainties, and low self-esteem, they also spoke about the
satisfaction when they were able to recognize a potential difficulty before it was apparent through the regular diagnostic channels associated with hospital technology, or the value of their
nurturant activities despite the devaluing of this by a society
interested in dramatic cures. The following account is typical of
the transformative actions in which nurses engage as a consequence of their intuition combining powers of observation,
which detects minute changes before they are evident, with their
nursing knowledge, clinical experience, and relational skills.

> I was working as a senior nurse on night duty in the
> neonatal intensive care. A new baby was admitted. He

was an FLK, which means he was a funny looking kid in the sense that he appeared as if he may have had some kind of genetic abnormality, some kind of syndrome which as yet hadn't been identified. The doctor who admitted him was very "ho hum" routine about it and just set up the normal things such as IV, nil orally, and put him into an Isolette, with some oxygen. He was allocated to a junior nurse. I was looking after the baby in the adjourning Isolette, and I kept an eye on this baby as he didn't look right to me. I wasn't sure if that was just because he was a FLK. The junior nurses kept asking me for help with his care. I had a good look at the baby and wasn't happy with him. After some time he seemed to be getting increasing respiratory distress, so I went to see the nurse in charge and told her that the baby didn't look good and suggested that we get the doctor back. It was about 1 a.m., and she didn't want to ring the doctor because she knew he was asleep downstairs. I told her that he was paid to be on call and to respond to our calls. She suggested that we just do what he had ordered and that he would see the baby in the morning. She would never do anything unless a doctor ordered it, and she never challenged them about anything.

I went back and over the next few hours I kept monitoring that baby really closely. The junior nurse and I tried everything; we suctioned out his airways; we repositioned him every which way; we kept listening to his chest; we tried different oxygen levels and still he didn't look right, but it wasn't really obvious, and I kept thinking it may not be an potential emergency, it may be just some unusual syndrome. I kept pestering the nurse in charge to get the doctor, but she said that we didn't have anything definite to wake him up for. At about 5 a.m. when I showed him that his blood pressure was lower, she agreed that I could phone the doctor. The doctor was pretty slack and asked me what I wanted him to do. I told him to come and check out this baby, and so he came and ordered some tests. It turned out that the baby had a cardiac lesion which this doctor had missed when he admitted him. The baby had a bowel obstruction as well and ended up being rushed off for surgery.

The clinical expertise of this nurse, her ability to assess the capacities of other staff and her perseverance on behalf of a baby who was not really her responsibility, saved the life of this child. This nurse's confidence in her gut feelings had developed over time as she cared for very ill babies.

Nurses also reported feelings of identification with patients who were being oppressed by the hospital system because of their own experiences within the system. Nurses regularly complained about hospital food and so often worked hard to get special delicacies or particular foods to entice patients to eat. The commonality of their experience of hospital food enabled them to appreciate patient difficulties.

Embodiment as Limit

As previously argued, nurses are embodied people whose habitual bodily patterns and routines cause them to act in particular ways. At times during the research when I had discussed rational transformative actions with a group of nurses and we had agreed that a particular action would be liberating, then someone would say, "I know that it is right and rational, but I know I just won't be able to do it because when X happens I always do Y; I can't help myself." Then the others would agree. These bodily patterns, which belong to nursing culture, are so enscribed on the bodies of people who have been nurses that many years after nurses have stopped nursing they report that they continue to engage in habitual actions from their nursing days and recognize other nurses by these habitual body responses. Nurses claimed that their bodies continue to act and react in habitualized and routinized patterns, which did not change even when the nurse made a rational decision to change. It was quicker and less stressful for nurses to continue to allow their bodies to work in ritualized ways than to act independently on the basis of a conscious decision, even when those actions could be demonstrated to contribute to the maintenance of technologies of power that were oppressive.

Lack of Clarity and Lack of Consensus

Rational change is also limited by a lack of clarity and consensus concerning nursing goals. Nursing has become a generalist label for a cluster of increasingly specialized nursing roles. The push to specialization has left many nurses feeling ill-equipped to work in any area other than their specialization. As this trend enlarges nurses are developing specialist jargon, procedures and processes relating to their specialties, but these groups of new knowledge and expertise serve to alienate nurses from the knowledge and expertise of other nurses. Correspondingly nurses are becoming distanced from the hopes and aspirations of other nurses in different areas. The rapid change to tertiary education and the influence of different disciplines on nursing scholars has served to separate the aspirations of the articulate voices of nursing from the clinical nurses they represent. According to Diane:

> ...the educators and administrators are only there as a service to the clinical practitioners, and yet the balance of power is quite, quite the opposite. They would never consider us first.

Role Confusion and Deskilling

Neither academic nurses nor nursing union representatives are able to reach a rational concensus on nursing goals with each other or within their own groups. Although they can identify issues, their espoused responses support particular ideological and professional interests that are at variance with the variety of issues and goals pursued by clinical nurses. The nurses in the research were atypical in the respect that they were prepared to use free time outside of their work hours to investigate their clinical practice and the values implicit in it. On broad issues they presented a similar capacity to critique nursing, however, nurses in the exploratory and pilot phases provided a much wider diversification in the range of their responses to questions about their goals and aspirations as nurses. The range of understandings and commitments to nursing and their roles as nurses was exacerbated by the large number of nurses who work part time. Many women who work only one shift per week in the same ward at the same time, or who work regular shifts in a particular area, expressed real concern about the trends being posed by nursing academics. These women did not want large changes to nursing because they will be deskilled. The issue of deskilling is a vital one in nursing with its increased emphasis on specializations and the need for increased technological competence. During the research I encountered nurses who were excited about their technological expertise and argued that greater technical and management training was empowering for nursing. However, many others were very anxious that they were being deskilled, and the values that they hold as practical, caring nurses were being devalued. It was apparent that nurses were unable to agree on goals for nursing because different value stances produced different rationally defensible positions.

The Freedom/Happiness Dichotomy in Clinical Practice

Nursing autonomy is a position argued theoretically by academics, administrators, union officials, and some clinical nurses. However, there is not necessarily a correlation between freedom and happiness. Nurses who value the nurturant aspect of their role and find happiness within it might express concern that a power/knowledge critique might enable them to identify and act upon their oppression but might not bring them happiness because their experiences of happiness in nursing have been formed historically by their negotiation of nursing culture. Many discussions with nurses about their experiences of making a difference in the lives of their patients were related to activities and relationships that were nurturant but not necessarily liberating for them personally. Busy nurses fought for nonnursing duties in order to free them from some of the routinized tasks related to patient care. However, the consequences have not always proved to provide happiness or good patient care because nurses adopt a role of relying on others for information about their patients in the same way as they critique doctors for relying on them. Comments from nurses reflected the consequences of this freedom from non-nursing duties for the patients and for themselves:

> I am glad we don't have to clean the pans or tidy the linen cupboard, but I am really sorry about the tasks which we have handed over to untrained staff which have to do with our patients. Now they are the ones who know if the patient has eaten their food or not, but they are not trained to understand the consequence of that knowledge. I like to know how much patients ate and what they had and why they didn't eat particular things. Now because I

don't give out or collect food trays I often don't get a chance to really check on the patient's likes and dislikes or the balance of their diet and think about it in light of my overall knowledge of the patient. The same is true about flowers. Before I used to talk about them with the patient as I put them in water, and I would learn about their visitors, and sometimes they would open up and say things that were important to their happiness and well-being. Now, I have to remember to go and comment later, but it will be the ward assistant who will have been told the important information. (RN, surgical ward)

Lately I've been following the meals lady around, which seems stupid as it doubles my work, but two weeks ago we had a problem. One of our male diabetics, who was very (medically) unstable, told the meals attendant that he didn't like a particular dessert, and so she swapped it with another patient who was happy about the swap. However, we didn't know, and later he went into a coma, and I couldn't understand his symptoms because I knew he was on a special sugarless diet. It wasn't until later that we learned what had happened. I felt really frustrated. It is difficult, too, when you have to find the staff or else ask patients how much fluid they had consumed. The staff often don't remember, and the patient may get confused or deliberately tell you the wrong thing because they want to go home or something. (RN, medical ward)

Autonomy is not generally a concept tied with motherhood, but although nurses did not want to continue to play mother to the doctors' "father," many expressed that they found happiness and gratification from bringing the fruits of their experiences of mothering or being mothered, to patient care and staff relations. Although highly critical of the double burden she and others experience of being female and being a nurse in a hierarchical, male-dominated medical system, Carol describes herself as an "earth mother" and her role as maternalistic.

My approach is maternalistic. When I know that trouble is brewing, I say to my staff "we are not going well," and we go into the back room and have a grudge session. The problems are aired, and we usually end up in fits of laughter. The kind of problems that surface in these sessions are "I am sick to death of handover starting at 7:10 when it is supposed to start at 7." If we have had patients that pose problems for the nurses on the ward such as a young patient dying, then we all sit down together and I pass the tissues...With some staff members you can see that they have lots of resentment from their displays of body language. I usually approach the person and say "I get the feeling that you are not happy, if the problem is personal then let's leave it, but if it is something related to the ward then let's talk about it." Then we can talk it through.

It is apparent that Carol's brand of maternalism is empowering for her staff. She engages in nurturant activities, which inform her clinical knowledge and form the basis for changed action.

Since the RANF strike many nurses have been uncomfortable with the direction taken by the radical nurses who were leading their fight for professional wages and nursing autonomy. During the November 1988 election of RANF officers, the entire team of twenty-two radical left-wing nursing unionists who had been actively responsible for the 1986 strike were replaced by a moderate center-wing faction. The previous team with its high proportion of clinical nurses has been replaced by a team headed by nursing administrators and educators. This voting pattern suggests that Victorian nurses have decided that continued strike action towards professional autonomy is not consistent with their happiness and that the loss of self-respect and respect from their patients, the general public, and the medical profession during and after the strike was a higher price than they are prepared to pay at present.

Nurturance/Knowledge as Emancipatory Knowledge

Feminist critical theorists have challenged the power/knowledge focus because they argue that it represents a male worldview, which is treated as gender-neutral, therefore obliterating the distinctive female power of nurturance (Balbus 1987). It was apparent from the data collected in this study that the power/knowledge orientation is limiting and that nurturance/knowledge is also a powerful orientation capable of leading to enlightenment, empowerment, and emancipation.

Nurses engaged in numerous instances of practice that transformed the situation for their patients from a basis of nurturance/knowledge. In the process of these engagements in transformative action, the nurses acted in ways that challenged the hegemony of the power structures adding to their own enlightenment and empowerment. In the following account it is evident that the nurse engaged in transformative action from a position of nurturance/knowledge:

> I was on night duty in ICU and when I arrived at the handover room at the beginning of the shift I noticed two very distressed parents. I overheard the evening shift charge nurse telling the night duty charge nurse that they had some "problem" parents. I thought to myself "I bet I get their baby." Handover progressed, and the charge nurse talked about this 16-month-old baby who had been rushed to casualty at another hospital after a cot death and been revived. The doctors had fussed around deciding whether to resuscitate, but the parents wanted them to go ahead. The baby revived but was not in good shape, and I guess they didn't know what to do with him next, so he was transferred to our ICU. Our specialist had examined him and pronounced him brain dead, and the doctor was trying to calm the parents to talk about it to them. This was one week after I had been to a lecture on brain death, and I remembered the doctor telling us to watch for a warm body with a cold head. Well, as I had anticipated the charge nurse gave me the baby to look after, and as I trotted down to the room all I could think of was, "Oh no I can't, I want to be sick." All through the bedside handover from the other nurse I had the thought running through my mind "warm body, cold head," and as soon as I finished checking the equipment and the procedures I put my hand on his head and thought, "oh no it's like a bag of frozen peas from the freezer." The doctor had told the parents that he would not do any more to the boy because of the long time he had been clinically dead before resuscitation, but naturally they were still very distressed. My role was to give the baby general nursing care and maintain the life support systems. I began looking after him, and as I gave him general nursing care I looked at this beautiful child and I thought, "if this was my child what would I want to do?" I talked to

the parents about him, asking them about what kind of boy he was and what he liked doing. As they talked about him they became much calmer, and I talked about his medical problems. We talked for about an hour, and they understood that he was going to die. I thought if this was my child, I wouldn't want him to die connected to all this equipment. He had no blood pressure to speak of, and so I asked if they would like to cuddle him. Of course they wanted to, and so, as the doctor had disappeared, I took him off the ventilator and gave him to his mother. I gave him a re-breathing bag attached to an tube so that I was legally covered by maintaining his airway and giving oxygen, but that wasn't really helping to prolong life like the ventilator does. Their relatives arrived, and they all sat and held the baby. We just sat and talked and talked and did lots of grieving, and I thought, "if this was me, this is what I would want." This went on for about an hour and a half until the baby died. I called the doctor and told him what I had done. He was grateful and let me take out the baby's tubes although for the autopsy you are supposed to send them off to the mortuary with all their tubes. I cleaned up the baby, and I took him and the parents to a little side room. They sat together cuddling the baby for about two hours and we talked over everything until they finally felt able to leave their baby. I cut a snippet of his hair for them to keep, and I organized to get his rug sent from the other hospital for them to keep. I just kept thinking, "if this was me, how would I want to be treated in this situation."

In this incident the nurse acted as the midwife for the grieving process. She demonstrated her capacity to ignore her initial feelings of fear and revulsion at caring for the brain dead child and to focus on using her personal and professional knowledge to engage in a process of intersubjective relationship with the parents and family. This process of making meanings out of the intersubjective relationship developed a commitment to their best interests. She reflected on her knowledge of herself, on the situation, and on her capacity to change the situation. This led to enlightenment about the situation, which showed her that she had the power to choose to maintain the baby and the situation or to deliberately choose to be proactive by initiating a situation, which was technically

beyond her proscribed power as a nurse but which was important to her ethics as a caring person. In her actions she collaborated with the parents in empowering them to make decisions
about their grieving process and the manner in which their
baby was to die. However, her constant support and nurturance of the whole family was based on her clinical experiences
of caring for other dying people and their relatives and in turn
affirmed and developed her knowledge of this nursing process.
She was accountable to the parents and to the doctor and was
prepared to defend her own actions because of their consistency with her espoused values of caring. Her reflections on her
values and the subsequent translation of those values into
action transformed the situation for everyone.

As nursing moves to more holistic understandings of
health and death as patterns of life, nurses can begin to place
their nursing knowledge into action that is empowering and
transforming for their patients, their colleagues, and themselves.

14

❦

Everyone Knows That!

The discipline of nursing, like any discipline, holds shared common meanings concerning taken-for-granted knowledge about how things are understood and done. These meanings make up what it means to be a nurse and, therefore, powerfully and profoundly penetrate nursing culture.

Nursing as a Culture of Unspoken Values

The culture of clinical nursing is an uncharted map of nursing care in which the values of clinical nurses are taken-for-granted and, therefore, are not always evident in the values espoused by nursing leaders. Although some of these values are revealed when the power/knowledge grid is placed over the map of nursing care, others are hidden further and only become evident when a nurturance/knowledge grid is used.

The Unspoken Values of an Oral Nursing Culture

Power/knowledge can demonstrate the ways in which the oral basis of nursing culture causes nurses to continue to be oppressed because they are unable to move from individualism to collaboration, they are unable to document their clinical knowledge and practice for reflection and critique, and they are unable to challenge the power base of the medical and administrative cultures articulated and perpetuated through means of written communication.

Perry (1987) and other nurse scholars argue that clinical

nurses remain unempowered in an oral culture when they are unable to articulate their knowledge and expertise to colleagues, doctors, and administrators through the permanency of written forms of communication or to to document it for their own reflective processes. The reluctance of clinical nurses to develop the skills necessary to communicate and receive knowledge through written forms gives them less access to the channels of power, which, by consequence, restricts and shapes their knowledge and their capacity to facilitate change. The work of Benner (1984:8) argues the necessity for nurses to record their clinical practice in order to uncover the meanings and expertise inherent in it. Other nurse scholars argue that documentation provides the means by which nurses can challenge the medical/gender domination of nursing by the medical and administrative cultures.

These arguments are rationally defensible if the value of a culture based on written communication is legitimated over an orally based culture. However, clinical nurses have consistently resisted developing nursing as a culture based on written practices. Nurses who have moved from clinical practice into administrative positions expend a deal of energy directed at the development of the recording skills and practices of clinical nurses. At the same time they support and maintain the oral culture of nursing through structural practices such as the oral handover and the double shift time. These double standards provide mixed messages to clinical nurses and reflect a biculturalism in which administrators recognize the value of oral practices at the same time as they recognize the value of nursing records for the development of nursing and the protection of patients.

This biculturalism of nursing administrators has developed because they are able to recognize the limitations of the oral culture for the development of the discipline of nursing and for the development of the knowledge and skills of practitioners. They recognize that the oral basis of nursing culture does not facilitate in nurses the capacity to systematically record and analyze their practice. Their response is to attempt to develop a written culture which coexists with the oral culture. It would appear from the observations and discussions throughout this research that the constant and continuing resistance, to administrative attempts to introduce a coexistent written nursing culture to the oral base of nursing, represents a counterhegemonic movement by clinical nurses. This resistance is never formally organized but constitutes part of the "common-sense" knowledge of what it means to be a nurse. Nurses "know" that the recorded data is "a waste of time" and so passively resist by either avoidance or through deliberately ineffective records. The unspoken value of this aspect of clinical practice is the valuing of the development of oral skills. Clinical nurses emphasized again and again that their interests lay in providing quality care, and that nursing academics and administrators appeared to them to be more interested in the recorded care than in the actual care.

A nurturance/knowledge grid placed over the map of nursing care would begin with a premise that the expressive capacity of oral communication leads to knowledge development, which is passed on and developed orally through a number of structures. This premise values the intersubjective meanings within the relationships in which nurses engage continually with visitors, patients, and staff and rejects the need for written records for the development of nursing knowledge and skills. The valuing of the oral culture of nursing would challenge the legitimation of the written cultures of the male-dominated medical and administrative cultures and actively support the further development of the kind of descriptive and expressive oral skills, which are generally the domain of women.

Legitimation of an oral nursing culture would only be possible if the challenges of nursing oppression exposed through ideology critique were addressed. My personal experiences of taping oral conversations with nurses for analysis and reflection demonstrated the sophistication of their skills of memory, description, and analysis. Although these women were not confident of their skills of writing about nursing practice, I found that that they were highly articulate concerning their views about themselves, their nursing practices, and nursing issues. They were capable of maintaining continuity of thought despite constant interruptions and of constructing telling arguments or critiques through conversation.

The work of feminist social researchers demonstrates that it is possible to value the oral culture, which supports the socializing and enculturing processes of our communal life, and to value both the nurturant activities in which women in particular engage and the knowledge which develops from and informs them (Oakley 1986). Feminists have shown that it is possible to develop structures, such as consciousness-raising groups, which are explicitly political in intent and content, in order to explicate the political implications of personal decisions. In other words women learn to value their culture through collaborative retelling of their experiences and knowledge and by researching their histories to challenge the ideologies that have devalued them. These oral processes have been supported through the work of feminist social researchers who have developed strategies for the compilation and analysis of women's oral histories (McRobbie 1982). This recording has been essential for the process of critique and affirmation of hitherto unspoken values.

The valuing of these unspoken values that support the oral culture of nursing would need to provide mechanisms by which this oral culture can be easily preserved for knowledge generation and analysis. Structural mechanisms would be essential to support developments such as groups designed to critique hegemonic structures and false consciousness. Audio and visual data collection techniques would need to be implemented alongside other orally based data collection systems such as voice-activated computers, which are capable of storing and producing printouts of nursing discussions, handovers, care plans, nursing notes, and descriptive accounts of practice. However, these structures would need to be developed collaboratively with clinical nurses, in order that their transformative potential is not reduced to another insidious form of surveillance. A serious examination, which poses problems and facilitates collaborative discourse and action, is necessary. This collaboration would aim to enhance and value the oral culture of nursing while meeting the needs of the administrators, and the clinical nurses themselves, for information on nursing practices as a basis for enlightenment, empowerment, and transformative action.

This process of empowerment of clinical nurses requires that they are able to challenge the bases of their adherence to the oral culture in the light of the legitimation of the written medical and administrative cultures. At present nurses adhere to an unspoken valuing of their oral culture through knowledge and experience while devaluing it through their unexamined support for the legitimizing practices of the recorded medical and administrative cultures. Clinical nurses experience the oral practices that constitute the oral basis of nursing as positive and enhancing, but rather than challenging the legitimacy of the data collection strategies being developed by educators and administrators, these nurses continue to engage in counterhegemonic practices, which resist the imposition of new practices without actually empowering themselves or their patients in the process. Nurses need to collaboratively examine the basis of their oral culture and consciously engage in structured emancipatory actions that bring enlightenment to, and transformation for, their patients. Nurses need to move from a position of passive resistance to a proactive position, which examines the values of data collection strategies and acts to develop positive strategies to document researchable descriptive data for analysis. This action is essential if nurses are to be able to systematically develop knowledge from practice, share that knowledge with others, and use that knowledge to improve the quality of care provided for their patients.

The Unspoken Values of Temporality

A power/knowledge focus reveals those aspects of nursing culture that are constrained by temporality. A power/knowledge analysis reveals the rigidity of ordering of work times and shifts and the manner by which nurses are oppressed by these structures. Nurses rapidly learn that they have limited time within any shift to achieve all the tasks allocated to them and to be able to deal with emergencies. This emphasis oppresses nurses by creating regular stress related to the organization of their work load. Nurses experience constant stress caused by the need to complete tasks, to cope with emergencies, and to relate to patients. It appears that the capacity to organize tasks and the capacity to spend time in developing therapeutic relationships with patients are both unspoken values of nursing culture, which often causes dissonance for nurses. However, both of these values contribute to a valuing of problem solving. Nurses who are trained to respond rapidly and competently to emergencies develop a problem-solving "quick fix" response to both tasks and patient problems. The technical approach to problem solving has led nurses to value the application of knowledge to solve problems.

These problems are taken for granted, and nurses in the research assumed that they could then take the problem and apply their knowledge and experience to solve it. Power/knowl-

edge demonstrates the reproduction of power relations in problem-solving approaches that do not question the politics informing the questions. Reflection and ideology critique enables nurses to begin to pose new questions and reframe old questions in
new ways rather than relying on taken-for-granted questions
that maintain oppressive situations.

Nurturance/knowledge demonstrates that when nurses
are acting to transform the situation for their patients, they
often do create new questions but generally do not record the
consequences of the planned action as a basis for collaborative
analysis and knowledge building. These questions are unacknowledged and unexplored and, therefore, do not contribute
to the development of nursing knowledge.

The Unspoken Values of Medical Dominance

A power/knowledge grid uncovers aspects of medical
domination, which oppresses nurses and patients. The legitimation of medical knowledge, practices, and ethics entails a
concurrent devaluing of nursing knowledge, practices, and
ethics. Medical dominance perpetuates class-based rewards of
status, high economic renumeration, professional autonomy,
and state-supported spheres of influence over other related
health workers. Medical dominance enables doctors to develop
the cultural basis of health and illness through medical definitions, which become socially acceptable and are followed by
prescription and proscription by doctors. The consequence of
this dominance for nursing is a lack of professional autonomy
as work is subjugated to, and regulated by, doctors. Nurses
receive poor economic rewards for high-stress work and
achieve minimal status or influence. The subjugation of nurses
is perpetuated through the disadvantages of class and gender.
My observations would suggest that ancillary staff experience
this subjugation through class, gender, and ethnicity, whereas
patients in general hospitals experience medical domination by
class, gender, ethnicity, and age.

Although power/knowledge enables nurses to critique medical domination, nurturance/knowledge reveals the reciprocity
in relationships between medical and nursing staff and demonstrates that most nurses believe that most doctors do value
nursing knowledge and skill, even though they underestimate it
or judge it against their own needs and medical criteria. This was

particularly apparent in the areas of specializations such as neonatal pediatrics, critical care, obstetrics, and oncology, where nurses were more familiar than medical staff with the technology used and with the patterns of healing and dying through repeated exposure to these kinds of specific patients. In these areas nurses often suggested that they were a respected member of the team as medical staff took up their ideas, comments, and suggestions on behalf of patients. All the nurses in the study valued their participation in team relationships with doctors and found this team participation one of the rewarding aspects of their nursing. The nurturance/knowledge grid demonstrated the important role played by nurses in the doctor/nurse team through their skills of communication and intersubjective meaning making for patients and doctors. In general discussions some nurses were particularly vociferous in denouncing nurses who wanted to separate the nursing role from the medical role, claiming that they were "antidoctor and antimen" and wanted to make nursing into some isolated female profession. Although the nurses sometimes appeared to be powerless in my observations of their team interactions, they themselves perceived their situation differently because they experienced the interactive role as satisfying. The contestation and critique of these observations, and the meanings attributed to them by the nurses, revealed that the unspoken value by which nurses judged the team effectiveness was in terms of their capacity to collaborate with the medical staff to bring about the best result for the patient. A commitment to collaborative action that nurtured the capacities of their colleagues to bring about quality patient care was valued more highly than the competitiveness that I was disclosing through a power/knowledge analysis. Nurses who value collaboration and their roles as team facilitators more readily tolerate the power plays of doctors, recognizing the power games and ignoring them or changing the rules without attempting to resist them. This valuing of collaboration, and the capacity of nurses to develop intersubjective meanings within team relationships that enhance patient care, is overlooked in an analysis based on power and interests. Any analysis of the doctor/nurse relations needs to recognize the transformative actions that can occur even in situations where nurses are oppressed and recognize that the limits to freedom experienced by nurses can contribute to their satisfaction and well-being because nursing culture values collaborative relationships over individual power positions.

The Unspoken Values of Nursing Role and Autonomy

A power/knowledge analysis of clinical nursing autonomy reveals the ways in which the nursing role ties nurses to shift work and to a role conducted at the bedside. By contrast doctors are seen to work in much more flexible ways and to be free to move throughout wards and other hospital areas. Nurses complain about their shifts and the inflexibility of their routines. However, it is apparent from nursing actions that nurses value their interpreting role, which emerges from the condition of being "tied to the bedside." The situation in which nurses are powerless to move away from the patient and their demands defines and shapes the nursing role so that nurses become patient-focused and develop a role as interpreter, coordinator, facilitator, and advocate on behalf of their patients. Nurses are able to engage in transformative action by virtue of their constant interaction with the patient. Therefore, nurses play lip service to challenges to the freedom and mobility of the medical staff while holding an unspoken value that supports the nurturance capacities of the bedside role and denigrates the medical mobility, which means that the doctor "knows" the patient mostly through the charts and the nurse's impressions.

Power/knowledge also demonstrates the way in which a commitment to objectivity within the nursing role oppresses nurses and patients. Shifts are organized so that nurses do not have successive shifts with the same patient. The patient and their relatives are oppressed by this system when they have to repeatedly relate intimate parts of their life story to strangers, particularly when the nurse they confided in yesterday is clearly visible in an adjourning section. Nurses are unable to pursue transformative action over time if they are expected to constantly relate to a new patients each shift. In this way nurses are robbed of the opportunity to work with patients to construct joint health goals and to work together to facilitate them. This lack of continuity militates against the capacity for nurses to research their own practice through reflection on strategic actions. In response to this limitation nurse scholars are developing strategies to enable nurses to engage in primary patient care where the responsibility for a patient is sustained over their entire stay in hospital.

This power/knowledge analysis and its subsequent empowering processes are resisted by clinical nurses who claim that these measures may not empower either the nurse or the patient. They suggest that it is unfair for nurses to have to provide continuous care for difficult or "heavy" patients over successive days. Others claim that their stress levels rise and they lose their capacity to think critically and creatively if they have too much exposure to patients who are emotionally exhausting. All the nurses in intensive care preferred looking after conscious patients, but each one suggested at times they found it so emotionally draining that they were glad to be allocated an unconscious patient whom they could care for without taxing their emotions in the way that happens with conscious patients.

The Unspoken Values of Nursing Resistance

Power/knowledge enables a process of ideology critique, which exposes the points of fragility in the structuring processes of hegemony in which resistance is possible or is active. Resistance in clinical nursing is strongest at the points where nurses believe that the best interests of individual patients are being overlooked, particularly when the unacknowledged ethics of nurses conflict with medical or administrative decisions and decision-making processes. Passive resistance occurs at points where the nursing culture designates that practices are inappropriate or unnecessary, such as the resistance to competency in written recording or the avoidance of medically or administratively derived tasks or decisions. Ideology critique reveals the technologies of power designed to produce docile nurses. However, this docility is partial as nurses respond through nurturance/knowledge to the intersubjective relationships with their colleagues and patients. These responses represent those acts of resistance that are shaped by the knowledge and experiences of clinical nursing care and are revealed in actions that transform the situations for others. Nurses discussing these acts of resistance recognize the reciprocity in the relationships and the contributions made to their own personal and professional growth and knowledge. Nursing resistance, which is based on a power/knowledge analysis, may be ultimately rejected if it causes nurses to experience too much dissonance with their personal and professional self-image of themselves as "caring" people. The self-image of caring person, which is supported by the values of clinical nursing culture, is reinforced through the positive experiences of nurturance activity.

A Critical Pedagogy for Nursing

Nurses are in the business of transforming lives through participation in the transformative healing/dying processes. Therefore, the emancipatory focus of critical pedagogy has an important contribution to make to the development of clinical nursing practices, which are transformative. A power/knowledge analysis enables nurses to develop critical theorems about their nursing practice, but this study demonstrated that the power/knowledge focus neglected the emancipatory nursing knowledge that develops from the experience of engaging in nursing care, which is essentially nurturant.

The combination of a power/knowledge analysis with a nurturance/knowledge analysis enables nurses to engage in an ideology critique, which reveals the unspoken values of clinical nursing practice for contestation and reconstruction. These analyzes and critiques will enable nurses to recognize the politics that constrain and oppress their clinical practices and to understand the mechanisms that maintain and legitimate oppressive structures for themselves and their patients.

This process of enlightenment requires that nurses participate in systematic learning processes of reflection and collaborative critique of their nursing actions, their sociocultural context, and the knowledge that informs and develops from these reflective processes. Collaborative discourse enables nurses to utilize the skills of their oral culture to engage in ideology critique and to plan systematic counterhegemonic actions, which empower their patients, their colleagues, and themselves. Other critical research methodologies such as journaling, critical case studies, critical ethnographies, action research, and critical clinical supervision could provide individuals and groups of nurses with the processes by which they can engage in their own enlightenment and empowerment. These processes need to be structured into the nursing culture by clinical nurses and not imposed from above or outside, although all the nurses in the study suggested that an outsider to the situation could facilitate these research-based processes in a way that enabled nurses to break the habits of horizontal violence and to collaborate together in critique, action, and reflection. This is essential if nurses are to move beyond the idiosyncratic and individualized focus of their transformative nursing practices and to work together to develop clinical nursing knowledge that is emancipatory and empowering.

Bibliography

Allen, D. G. "Nursing research and social control: Alternative Models of Science that emphasize understanding and emancipation." *Image: The journal of Nursing Scholarship* 17, no. 2 (Spring 1985): 58–64.

Alschuler, A. S. "Creating a world where it is easier to love: Counselling applications of Paulo Freire's theory." *Journal of Counselling and Development* 64 (April 1986): 492–96.

Anyon, Jean. "Intersections of gender and class: Accommodation and resistance by working-class and affluent females to contradictory sex role ideologies." *Journal of Education* 166, no. 1 (1984): 29–48.

Anzaldua, Gloria. "Haciendo caras, una entrada." In Gloria Anzaldua (ed.) *Making Face, Making Soul.* San Francisco: Aunt Lute Foundation Books, 1990, xv–xxviii.

Ashley, Jo Ann. "Power in structured misogyny: Implications for the politics of care." *Advances in Nursing Science* 2 (April 1980): 3–22.

Ashley, Jo Ann. *Hospitals, Paternalism and the Role of the Nurse.* New York: Teacher's College Press, Columbia University, 1972.

Bailey, J. T., and Claus, K. E. *Decision Making in Nursing.* St. Louis: The C. V. Mosby Co., 1975.

Balbus, Isaac D. "Disciplining women." In S. Benhabib and D.Cornell (eds.), *Feminism as Critique.* Cambridge: Polity Press, 1987.

Barclay, L. "Diploma of Applied Science (Nursing) Reaccreditation Research." Unpublished report of findings, S.A.C.A.E., 1986.

Benjamin, M., and Curtis, J. "Virtue and the practice of nursing," in E. Shelp (ed.), *Virtue and Medicine.* Boston: D. Reidel Publishing Company, 1985.

Benner, Patricia. *From Novice to Expert: Excellence and Power in Clinical Nursing Practice.* California: Addison-Wesley Publishing Company, 1984.

Benner, Patricia and Wrubel, Judith. *The Primacy of Caring.* California: Addison-Wesley Publishing Company, 1988.

Benoliel, J. "Scholarship—A women's perspective." *Image* 7, no. 2 (1975): 22–27.

Berlak, Ann. "Back to Basics: Liberating Pedagogy and the Liberal Arts." Paper presented to the Annual Meeting of the American Educational Research Association, Chicago, 1985.

Bernstein, Richard. *Beyond Objectivism and Relativism: Science, Hermeneutics and Praxis.* Philadelphia: University of Pennsylvania Press, 1983.

Bernstein, Richard. *The Restructuring of Social and Political Theory.* Philadelphia: University of Pennsylvania Press, 1978.

Bodemann, Y. M. "A problem of sociological praxis: The case for interventive observation in field work," *Theory and Society* 5, no. 3 (1978): 387–420.

Bordo, Susan R. "The Body and the Reproduction of Femininity: A feminist Appropriation of Foucault," in Alison M Jagger and Susan R Bordo, *Gender/Body/Knowledge,.* New Brunswick: Rutgers University Press, 1989

Boud, David (et al.). *Reflection: Turning Experience into Learning.* London: Kogan Page/New York: Nichols Publishing Company, 1985.

Brewer, Ann M. "Nurses, nursing and new technology: Implications of a dynamic technological environment." *Australian Studies in Health Service Administration* 47 (1986).

Bullough, Bonnie. "Barriers to the nurse practitioner movement: Problems of women in a woman's field,." *International Journal of Health Services* 5, no. 2 (1975): 225–33.

Bullough, R. (et al.). "Ideology, teacher role and resistance." *Teachers College Record* 86, no. 2 (1984): 339–58.

Burbules, Nicholas. "A theory of power in education." *Educational Theory* 36, no. 2 (Spring 1986).

Carper, Barbara A. "Fundamental patterns of knowing in nursing." *Advances in Nursing Science* 1 (Oct. 1978): 13–23.

Carr, Wilfred, and Kemmis, Stephen. *Becoming Critical: Knowing Through Action Research.* Victoria: Deakin University Press, 1983.

Chapman, C. M. "Concepts of professionalism." *Journal of Advanced Nursing* 2, no. 1 (1977): 51–55.

Chaska, Norma. *The Nursing Profession: A Time To Speak.* New York: McGraw-Hill Book Company, 1983.

Chaska, Norma. *The Nursing Profession: Views through the Mist.* New York: McGraw-Hill Book Company, 1978.

Chinn, Peggy and Wheeler, Charlene E. "Feminism and nursing." *Nursing Outlook* 33, no. 2 (1985): 74–77.

Cleland, Virginia. "Sex discrimination: Nursing's most pervasive problem." *American Journal of Nursing* 71 (1971): 1542–47.

Connell, Robert W. *Ruling Class, Ruling Culture.* Great Britain: Cambridge University Press, 1977.

Connell, Robert W. *Gender and Power.* Sydney: Allen and Unwin, 1987.

Cox, Helen, and Moss, Cheryle. "Promiscuous Knowledge—The Chaos of Practice." Conference Proceedings, International Nursing Conference: "Professional Promiscuity," Perth, December 1988,

Crowder, E. L. M. "Historical perspectives of nursing's professionalism." *Occupational Health Nursing* 33, no. 4 (1985): 184–90.

Daubenmire, J., and King, I. M. "Nursing Process Models: A Systems Approach." *Nursing Outlook* 21, no. 8 (1973): 512–17.

Davis, Mark, and Donohoe, Brendan. "Irene Bolger and the Cavaliers," in *The Age* 19/12/86.

Dickens, Charles. *Martin Chuzzlewit* Boston: Estes and Lauriat, 1896.

Dickoff, James, (et al.). "Theory in a practice discipline." *Nursing Research* 17, no. 5 (1968): 415–34.

Dimen, Muriel. "Power, Sexuality, and Intimacy," in Alison M. Jagger and Susan R. Bordo, *Gender/Body/Knowledge.* New Brunswick: Rutgers University Press, 1989

Dolan, Josephine A. *Nursing In Society: A Historical Perspective.* Philadelphia: W. B. Saunders Company, 1978.

Dreyfus, Stuart, E., and Dreyfus, Herbert L. "A Five-stage Model of the Mental Activities involved in Directed Skill Acquisition." Unpublished report supported by the Air Force Office of Scientific Research (AFSC), USAF (Grant AFOSR–78–3594), University of California at Berkeley, 1979.

Dreyfus, Herbert L. and Rabinow, Paul. *Michel Foucault: Beyond Struturalism and Hermeneutics.* Great Britain: The Harvester Press, 1982.

Dreyfus, Herbert L. "Holism and hermeneutics." *Review of Metaphysics* 34 (September 1980): 3–23.

Dunlop, Margaret J. "Is a science of caring possible?" *Journal of Advanced Nursing* 11 (1986): 661–70.

Ehrenreich, Barbara and English, Deidre. *Wives, Midwives and Nurses: A History of Women Healers.* New York: The Feminist Press, 1973.

Ehrenreich, John (ed.). *The Cultural Crisis of Modern Medicine.* New York: Monthly Review Press, 1978.

Eliot, T. S. *Four Quartets.* London: Faber and Faber, (rep.) 1986.

Etzioni, A. *The Semi-Professions and their Organization.* New York: The Free Press, 1969.

Evers, Helen. "Care or custody? The experiences of women patients in long-stay geriatric wards," in B. Hutter and G. Williams (eds.), *Controlling Women: The Normal and the Deviant.* London: Croom Helm, 1981.

Fawcett, J. "Hallmarks of success in nursing research." *Advances in Nursing Science* 7, no. 1 (1984): 1–11.

Fay, Brian. "How people change themselves: The relationship between critical theory and its audience," in T. Bull, (ed.), *Political Theory and Praxis: New Perspectives.* Minnesota: University of Minnesota Press, 1977.

Fay, Brian. *Critical Social Science.* Cornell Paperbacks, Cornell University Press, 1987.

Fay, Brian. *Social Theory and Political Practice.* London: Allen and Unwin, 1975.

Felman, Shoshana. *Jacques Lacan and the adventure of insight.* Cambridge, Massachusetts: Harvard University Press, 1987.

Foucault, Michel. *Discipline and Punish.* London: Penguin Books, 1975.

Foucault, Michel. *The Archeology of Knowledge and the Discourse of Language.* New York: Harper and Row, 1972.

Foucault, Michel. "Afterword: The subject and power," in L. Hubert D. and P. Rabinow (eds.), *Michel Foucault: Beyond Struturalism and Hermeneutics.* Great Britain: The Harvester Press, 1982.

Foucault, Michel. "Two lectures," in C. Gordon (ed.), *Power and Knowl-*

edge: Selected Interviews and Other Writings by Michel Foucoult, 1972–1977. New York: Pantheon, 1980(a).

Foucault, Michel. *The History of Sexuality, Volume 1: An Introduction.* New York: Vintage/Random House, 1980(b).

Fraser, Nancy. "What's critical about critical theory?" in S. Benhabib and D. Cornell, (eds.), *Feminism as Critique.* Cambridge: Polity Press, 1987.

Freire, Paulo. *The Politics of Education: Culture, Power and Liberation.* London: Macmillan, 1985.

Freire, Paulo. *Education for Critical Consciousness.* New York: Continuum, 1981.

Freire, Paulo. *Pedagogy of the Oppressed.* Harmondsworth: Penguin, 1972.

Friedan, Betty. *The Feminine Mystique.* England: Penguin, 1963.

Friedson, Eliot. *Profession of Medicine: A Study of the Sociology of Applied Knowledge.* New York: Dodd, Mead and Company, 1970.

Gadamer, Hans G. *Truth and Method.* New York: Seabury Press, 1975.

Game, Ann and Pringle, Rosemary, (eds.). *Gender At Work.* Sydney: George Allen and Unwin, 1983.

Gans, H. J. *The Levittowners.* New York: Random House Books, 1967.

Giddens, Anthony. *The Constitution of Society.* Cambridge: Polity Press, 1984.

Giroux, Henry. *Ideology, Culture and the Process of Schooling.* London: Falmer Press, 1981.

Giroux, Henry. "Curriculum study and cultural politics." *Journal of Education* 166, no. 3 (1984): 226–38.

Giroux, Henry. *Theory and Resistance in Education: A Pedagogy for the Opposition.* Massachusetts: Bergin and Garvey Publishers, 1983.

Giroux, Henry and McLaren, Peter. "Radical Pedagogy as Cultural Politics: Beyond the Discourse of Critique and Anti-Utopianism," in Donald Morton and Mas'ud Zavarzadeh (eds.) *Theory/Pedagogy/Politics.* Urbana, Champaign: University of Illinois Press, 1991, 152–86.

Glaser, B. G., and Strauss, A. L. *The Discovery of Grounded Theory.* Chicago: Aldine, 1967.

Gold, R. "Roles in sociological field observations." *Social Forces* 36 (1958): 217–23.

Gortner, Susan R. "The history and philosophy of nursing science and research." *Advances in Nursing Science* 5, no. 2 (1983): 1–8.

Gramsci, A. *Selections from the Prison Notebooks.* New York: International, 1971.

Greenleaf, N. F. "The sex segmented occupations: Relevance for nursing." *Advances in Nursing Science* 2 (April 1980): 23–37.

Grumperz, J. "Conversational inference and classroom Learning," in J. L. Green and C. Wallat (eds.), *Ethnography and Language in Educational Settings.* Norwood, New Jersey: Ablex, 1981.

Habermas, Jurgen. "Towards a theory of communicative competence." *Inquiry* 13, no. 4 (1970): 360–76.

Habermas, Jurgen. *Knowledge and Human Interests.* Boston: Beacon Press, 1971.

Habermas, Jurgen. *Theory and Practice.* Boston: Beacon Press, 1973(a).

Habermas, Jurgen. *Legitimation Crisis.* Boston: Beacon Press, 1973(b).

Hackett, Olive P. "Women and the health care system: A case study in feminist praxis." *Radical Religion* 3, no. 2 (1977): 36–43.

Hamilton, David. *In Search of Structure.* London: Hodder and Stoughton, 1977.

Hammersley, Martyn and Atkinson, Paul. *Ethnography: Principles in Practice.* London: Tavistock Publications, 1983.

Hartsock, Nancy C. M. *Money, Sex and Power.* New York: Longman, 1983.

Hedin, Barbara A. and Duffy, Mary E. "Researching: Designing Research from a Feminist Perspective," in proceedings from the conference, Caring and Nursing Explorations in the Feminist Perspectives, June 17–18 Denver, Colorado, 1988.

Heidegger, Martin. *Being and Time.* New York: Harper and Row, 1962.

Held, David. *Introduction to Critical Theory: Horkheimer to Habermas.* Berkeley: University of California Press, 1980.

Henderson, Virginia A. "Preserving the essence of nursing in a technological age." *Journal of Advanced Nursing* 5 (1980) 245–60.

Henderson, Virginia. "We've 'come a long way', but what of the direction?" *Nursing Research* 26, no. 3 (1977).

Henderson, Virginia. "The concept of nursing," in *Journal of Advanced Nursing* 3 (1978): 113–30.

Hirsch, Lolly. "Practicing health without a license," in K. Grimstad and S. Rennie (eds.), *The New Woman's Survival Sourcebook*. New York: Knopf, 1975.

hooks, bell. "Talking Back," in Russell Ferguson, Martha Gever, Trinh T. Minh-ha, and Cornel West (eds.) *Out There: Marginalization and Contemporary Cultures*. New York: The New Museum of Contemporary Art and Cambridge, Mass.: The MIT Press, 1990, 337–40.

Hunt, Maura. "The process of translating research findings into nursing practice." *Journal of Advanced Nursing* 12 (1987): 101–10.

Hymes, D. "What is ethnography?" *Sociolinguistic Paper* 45 (April 1978) Southwest Educational Development Laboratory, Texas.

Illich, Ivan (et al.). *Disabling Professions*. London: Marion Boyars, 1977.

Illich, Ivan. *Limits to Medicine*. London: Marion Boyars, 1976.

Infante, Mary S. "The clinical learning experience: The evolution of the nursing work force," in *National League for Nursing Patterns in Education: The Unfolding of Nursing*. New York, 1985.

Jennings, Leonie E. "Issues for Consideration by Case Study Workers." Paper presented at the Qualitative Symposium Research Network, Australian Association of Adult Education, North Ryde, May 1986.

Keen, Peggy. "Caring for each other," in proceedings from the conference, Caring and Nursing Explorations in the Feminist Perspectives, June 17–18, Denver, Colorado, 1988.

Kemmis, Stephen. "Action research and the politics of reflection," in D. Boud et al. (eds.), *Reflection: Turning Experience into Learning*. London: Kogan Page, and New York: Nichols Publishing Company, 1985.

Kenny, W. R. and Groteleuschen, A. "Making the case for case study." *Journal of Curriculum Studies* 16 (1984): 37–51.

Kubler-Ross, Elisabeth. *On Death and Dying*. New York: Macmillan, 1969.

Lacey, G. *Hightown Grammar.* Manchester: Manchester University Press, 1970.

Larson, M. S. *The Rise of Professionalism: A Sociological Analysis*. Berkeley: University of California Press, 1977.

Lather, Patti. "Research As Praxis." Unpublished paper presented at the Sixth Curriculum Theorizing Conference, Ohio, 1984(a).

Lather, Patti. "Critical theory, curricular transformation and feminist mainstreaming." *Journal of Education* 166, no. 1 (1984(b)).

Lather, Patti. "Empowering Research Methodologies." Unpublished paper to A.E.R.A., Chicago, 1985.

Lather, Patti. "Issues of Data Trutworthiness in Openly Ideological Research." Paper to American Educational Research Association, San Francisco, California, April 1986.

Leininger, M. (ed.). *Caring: An Essential Human Need.* Thorofare, N.J.: Charles B. Slack Inc., 1981.

Lemin, B. "The extended role of the nurse," in E. Jenkins (et al.) (eds.), *Issues in Australian Nursing.* Melbourne: Churchill Livingstone, 1982.

Lipman-Blumen, Jean. *Gender Roles and Power.* New Jersey: Prentice-Hall, 1984

Lofland, John. *Analyzing Social Settings: A Guide to Qualitative Observation.* California: Wadsworth, 1971.

Lovell, M. C. "The politics of medical deception: Challenging the trajectory of history." *Advances in Nursing Science* 2 (1980): 73–86.

Lutz, F. W. "Ethnography—The holistic approach to understanding schooling," in J. L. Green and C. Wallat (eds.), *Ethnography and Language in Educational Settings.* Norwood, New Jersey: Ablex, 1981.

Malinowski, B. *Argonauts of the Western Pacific.* London, 1922.

Mann, E. "New Strength," in Access Age, *The Age.* 19/11/86.

Maaresh, J. K. "Women's History, Nursing History: Parallel Stories." *Nursing and Feminism: Implications for Health Care.* New Haven: Yale University Press, 1986.

Marles, Fay (et al.). "Report of the Study of Professional Issues in Nursing," February 1988.

McCarthy, Thomas. *The Critical Theory of Jurgen Habermas.* Massachusetts: The MIT Press, 1985.

McLaren Peter. *Life in Schools.* New York: Longman, 1989.

McLaren, Peter. "Language, Social Structure and the Production of Subjectivity." *Critical Pedagogy Networker.* May/June 2 & 3:1–10, 1988a.

McLaren, Peter. "Schooling the Postmodern body; critical pedagogy and the politics of enfleshment." *Journal of Education*. vol. 170:53–83.1988b

McRobbie, Angela. "The politics of feminist research: Between talk, text and action." *Feminist Review* 12 October 1982.

Meleis, A. I. *Theoretical Nursing: Development and Progress*. Philadelphia: Lippincott, 1985.

Melosh, B. *"The Physician's Hand": Work Culture and Conflict in American Nursing*. Philadelphia: Temple University Press, 1982.

Menzies-Lyth, I. "Problems in the Health Services." A public lecture at the Victorian Hospitals Association, December 1986.

Mitchell, G. Duncan. *A Dictionary of Sociology*. London: Routledge and Kegan Paul, 1968.

Moccia, P. "A critque of compromise: beyond the methods debate." *Advances in Nursing Science* 10, no. 4 (1988): 1–9.

Monteiro, L. "Interdisciplinary stresses of extended nursing role," in N. Chaska (ed.), *The Nursing Profession: Views Through the Mist*. New York: McGraw-Hill Book Company, 1978.

Morgan, Robin. *Taking Back Our Bodies, The New Woman's Survival Sourcebook*. New York: Knopf, 1975.

Moss, Cheryle. "Portrait of a Nurse as a Practitioner." Proceedings of the Conference, "Courage To Learn," Austin Hospital, Melbourne, 1987.

Munhall, Patricia L. "Methodologic fallacies: A critical self-appraisal." *Advances in Nursing Science* 5 (July 1982): 41–49.

Nightingale, Florence. *Notes on Nursing*. London: Harrison and Sons, 1859 (Philadelphia: J. P. Lippincott Co., 1946).

O'Toole, Anita W. "When the practical becomes theoretical." *Journal of Psychiatric Nursing and Mental Health Studies* 19, no. 12 (December 1981): 11–16.

Oakley, Ann. "Interviewing women," in H. Roberts (ed.), *Doing Feminist Research*. London: Routledge and Kegan Paul, 1981.

Oakley, Ann. *Telling the Truth About Jerusalem*. London: Routledge and Kegan Paul, 1986.

Parker, Judith. "Theoretical Perspectives in Nursing: From Microphysics to Hermeneutics." *Shaping Nursing Theory and practice:*

The Australian Context. Monograph 1, Department of Nursing, Lincoln School of Health Sciences. La Trobe University, 1988.

Parse, Rosemary. *Man-Living-Health: A theory of nursing.* New York: John Wiley and Sons, 1981.

Pearsall, M. "Participant observation as role behaviour and method in behavioural research." *Nursing Research* 14, no. 1 (1965): 37–42.

Pearson, Alan. "Nurses as change agents and a strategy for change." *Nursing Practice* 2 (1985): 80–84.

Perry, Judith and Moss, Cheryle. "Generating Alternatives in Nursing: Turning Curriculum into a Living Process." *The Australian Journal of Advanced Nursing* 10, no. 4 (1988): 1–4

Perry, Judith. "Creating our own image." *NZ Nursing Journal,* February 1987: 10–13.

Perry, Judith. "Professional socialisation—A political process?" *Nursing Praxis in New Zealand* 1, no. 2 (March 1986).

Perry, Judith. "Creating Our Own Image." Unpublished paper to the conference Horizons of Care, N.Z. Nursing Education and Research Foundation, Wellington, 1985(b).

Perry, Judith. "Theory and Practice in the Induction of Five Graduate Nurses: A Reflexive Critique." Unpublished M.A. Thesis, Massey University, 1985(a).

Pittman, Elizabeth. "Goodbye Florence." *Australian Society* February 1985: 8–10.

Polanyi, M. *Personal Knowledge.* London: Routledge and Kegan Paul, 1962.

Polkinghorne, Donald *Methodology for the Human Sciences: Systems of Inquiry.* Albany: State University of New York Press, 1983.

Reeder, S. J. "The social context of nursing," in N. Chaska (ed.), *The Nursing Profession: Views Through the Mist.* New York: McGraw-Hill Book Company, 1978.

Reuther, Rosemary R. *New Woman New Earth: Sexist Ideologies and Human Liberation.* New York: Seabury Press, 1975.

Ricoeur, P. *Freud and Philosophy; an Essay on Interpretation.* Savage, D. (trans.). New Haven: Yale University Press, 1970.

Ricoeur, P. *Hermeneutics and the Human Sciences.* John Thompson (ed.). Cambridge: Cambridge University Press, 1981.

Roberts, Helen. *Doing Feminist Research.* London: Routledge and Kegan Paul, 1981.

Roberts, K. L. "Nursing: Profession or pretender?" *The Australian Nurses Journal* 9, no. 10 (1980): 33–51.

Roberts, S. J. "Oppressed group behaviour: Implications for nursing." *Advances in Nursing Science* July 1983: 21–30.

Rogers, Martha E. "Beyond the horizon," in N. Chaska (ed.), *The Nursing Profession: A Time to Speak.* New York: McGraw-Hill, 1981

Rogers, Martha E. "Nursing: The science of unitary man," in J. P.Riehl and C. Roy (eds.), *Conceptual models for Nursing Practice.* 2nd edition. Appleton-Century-Crofts, 1980.

Rogers, Martha E. "The nature and characteristics of professional education for nursing." *Journal of Professional Nursing* 1, no. 6 (1985): 381–83.

Rowbotham, Sheila. *Women's Consciousness, Man's World.* Harmondsworth: Penguin Books, 1973.

Roy, Sister Callista. "The Roy adaption model," in J. P. Riehl and C. Roy (eds.), *Conceptual Models for Nursing Practice,* 2nd ed. New York: Appleton-Century-Crofts, 1980.

Roy, Sister Callista. *Introduction to Nursing: An Adaption Model.* New Jersey: Prentice-Hall, 1981.

Ryan, William. *Blaming the Victim.* New York: Vintage Books, 1971.

Schön, Donald. *Educating the Reflective Practitioner.* San Francisco: Jossey Bass Publishers, 1987.

Schön, Donald. *The Reflective Practitioner: How Professionals Think in Action.* New York: Basic Books, 1983.

Schrag, C. O. *Communicative praxis and the space of subjectivity.* Bloomington: Indiana University Press, 1986.

Silva, M. C., and Robarth, D. "An analysis of changing trends in philosophies of science on nursing theory development and testing." *Advances in Nursing Science* 6, no. 2 (1984): 1–13.

Simms, L. M. "The grounded theory approach in nursing research." *Nursing Research* 30, no. 6 (1981): 356–59.

Simon, Roger I. "For a Pedagogy of Possibility." *Critical Pedagogy Networker* 1, no. 1: 1–4, Deakin University, 1988.

Smith, John. "Quantitative versus qualitative research: An attempt to clarify the issue." *Educational Researcher* 12, no. 3 (1983): 6–13.

Smith, Ruth. "Nurses' action involves more than wages," in Letters to the Age, *The Age.* 10 November 1986, p.12.

Speedy, Sandra. "Femininism and the professionalisation of nursing." *The Australian Journal of Advanced Nursing* 4, no. 2 (December 1986, February 1987).

Spender, Dale. "The gatekeepers: A feminist critique of academic publishing," in H. Roberts (ed.), *Doing Feminist Research.* London: Routledge and Kegan Paul, 1981.

Spradley, J. *The Ethnographic Interview.* New York: Holt, Rinehart and Winston, 1979.

Stein, L. "The nurse-doctor game." *Archives of General Psychiatry* 16 (1967): 699–703.

Stenhouse, Lawrence. "Case study methods." *International Encyclopaedia of Education.* London: Pergamon Press, 1985.

Street, Annette, *From Image to Action: Reflection in Nursing Practice.* Victoria: Deakin University Press, 1990

Styles, Margareta M. *On Nursing: Toward a New Endowment.* Missouri: C. V. Mosby Co., 1982.

Tandon, Rajesh. "Participatory research in the empowerment of people." *Convergence* 14, no. 3 (1981).

Thompson, Janine. "Practical discourse in nursing: Going beyond empiricism and historicism." *Advances in Nursing Science* 7, no. 4 (1985): 59–72.

Tiffany, R. "Nursing—Industry or profession?" *The Australian Nurses Journal* 11, no. 9 (1982): 43–45.

Tomich, J. H. "The expanded role of the nurse: Current status and future prospects," in N. Chaska (ed.), *The Nursing Profession: Views Through the Mist.* New York: McGraw-Hill Book Company, 1978.

Walker, R. "On the uses of fiction in educational research (and I don't mean Cyril Burt)," in *Case Study Methods.* Geelong: Deakin University, 1982.

Watson, J. "Nursing on the caring edge: metaphorical vignettes." *Advances in Nursing Science* 10, no. 1 (1987): 10–18.

Weber, M. *The Protestant Ethic and the Spirit of Capitalism.* London: Unwin University Books, 1965.

Weedon, C. *Feminist Practice and Poststructuralist Theory*. London: Basil Blackwell, 1987.

Wheeler, Charlene, E. and Chinn, Peggy L. *Peace and Power*. New York: National League for Nursing, 1989.

Whyte, W. E. *Street Corner Society: The Social Structure of an Italian Slum*. Chicago: University of Chicago Press, 1981.

Williams, Raymond. *Marxism and Literature*. Oxford: Oxford University Press, 1977.

Willis, Evan. *Medical Dominance*. Australia: George Allen and Unwin, 1983.

Willis, Paul. *Learning to Labor*. London: Saxon House, 1977.

Wilson, Stephen. "The use of ethnographic techniques in educational research." *Review of Educational Research* 47, no. 1 (1977): 245–65.

Winstead-Fry, M. "The Scientific Method and Its Impact on Holistic Health." *Advances in Nursing Science* 2 (1980): 1–9.

Wright, Peter W. G. "The radical sociology of medicine." *Social Studies of Science* 10, no. 1 (1981): 103–20.

Yeaworth, R. C. "Feminism and the nursing profession," in N. Chaska (ed.), *The Nursing Profession: Views Through the Mist*. New York: McGraw-Hill Book Company, 1978.

Yuen, F. "Multi-dimensional approach: A task for curriculum development." *Journal of Advanced Nursing* 12 (1987): 52–62.

Index